MALE TROUBLE

MALE TROUBLE
A New Focus on the Prostate

GILBERT CANT

A Frank E. Taylor Book

Praeger Publishers • New York

To my wife
who is fortunate to have
no prostate trouble

Published in the United States of America in 1976
by Praeger Publishers, Inc.
111 Fourth Avenue, New York, N.Y. 10003

© 1976 by Gilbert Cant

Library of Congress Cataloging in Publication Data

Cant, Gilbert.
Male trouble.

"A Frank E. Taylor book."
Includes index.
1. Prostate gland—Diseases. I. Title.
RC899.C32   616.6'5   75-14646

ISBN 0-275-56370-7

Printed in the United States of America

Contents

Acknowledgments

Many urologists and other physicians have given the author invaluable assistance, either through their printed works or viva voce *in generous interview time, in compiling the material for this book. The mother lode of basic information on the anatomy, pathology, and surgery of the prostate is* Urology, *edited by M. F. Campbell and J. Hartwell Harrison, 3rd ed., 1970 (W. B. Saunders Company). A most useful and up-to-date source of technical opinion is* The Urologic Clinics of North America, *Vol. 2, No. 1, February 1975 (Saunders). Several of the contributors to this symposium have given the author additional personal help. It would be both impossible and invidious to try to rank individual sources by the volume or value of the assistance they have given, so they are gratefully listed here in alphabetical order:*

Malcolm A. Bagshaw, M.D., Stanford University School of Medicine; Aaron Bendich, Ph.D., Sloan-Kettering Institute, New York City; William G. Cahan, M.D., Memorial Sloan-Kettering Cancer Center, New York City; George C. Cotzias, M.D.,

Memorial Sloan-Kettering Center; Nancy B. Cummings, M.D., National Institutes of Health; J. R. Herman, M.D., Albert Einstein College of Medicine, The Bronx, N.Y.; Harry W. Herr, M.D., Memorial Sloan-Kettering Cancer Center; Harold A. Lear, M.D., Mount Sinai Medical Center, New York City; Eugene McCarthy, M.D., New York Hospital-Cornell Medical Center; Edwin M. Meares, Jr., M.D., Tufts University-New England Medical Center, Boston; Erich Meyerhoff, Director, Cornell University Medical College Library; Gerald P. Murphy, M.D., D.Sc., Project Director, National Prostatic Cancer Project and Director, Roswell Park Memorial Institute, Buffalo, N.Y.; Philip R. Roen, M.D., New York Medical College, New York City; Jack Saroff, Ph.D., Roswell Park Memorial Institute; William Wallace Scott, M.D., Brady Urological Institute, Johns Hopkins Hospital, Baltimore, Md.; Thomas A. Stamey, M.D., Stanford University School of Medicine; Patrick C. Walsh, M.D., Professor and Director, Department of Urology, Johns Hopkins University School of Medicine; Willet F. Whitmore, Jr., M.D., Memorial Sloan-Kettering Cancer Center.

These sources are not to blame if the book suffers from errors of omission or commission; the full responsibility for these rests upon

THE AUTHOR.

Foreword

Every man has a prostate gland. About half of all men of European extraction, which include the majority of North Americans, are fortunate enough to remain happily unaware of it throughout their lives. But for the other half the prostate is the source and cause of a variety of disorders and diseases, some relatively minor and others of major importance. The great majority of these appear in the later years of a normal life span; because many more men are now reaching advanced ages, the number of cases of prostatic disorder is increasing proportionately. The average expectation of life for an American male has been extended within this century from a mere forty-nine years to almost exactly seventy. Today approximately 30 million men in the United States are in the most susceptible age group, forty-five and over. This means that 15 million of us will sooner or later suffer from a prostate disorder that may require medical attention. In Canada, with a population about one tenth that of the United States, the number will be one and a half million.

There are, incidentally, questions in regard to

racial susceptibility. Some recent studies indicate that there has been a sharper increase in prostatic disease and certainly in prostatic cancer among American blacks than among the white population. It is not certain whether this represents a true epidemiological phenomenon or whether it is a statistical artifact, because in recent years a much greater proportion of blacks have been obtaining better medical care than before. The difficulty of interpreting the statistics is heightened by the fact that most blacks in North America and some Caribbean islands are now of mixed blood. The island of Barbados, with a predominantly black population, relatively unmixed, supplies significant data. Of the forty-four nations in the world for which the American Cancer Society has reliable figures, Barbados ranks fourth for mortality from prostate cancer (after Sweden, Switzerland and Norway), with a far higher rate than that for the United States. On the other hand, prostate cancer is rare among Asians who remain in their native lands. The rate for North America is a hundred times as high as that for Japan. But when Asians migrate eastward, first to Hawaii and then to mainland America, their incidence of prostate disease increases. This cannot be genetic but must reflect a change in life style.

What we are observing is most emphatically not an epidemic comparable with the great plagues of history, but instead an apparently natural—if little understood—aspect of the aging process. Although only 50 percent of all men are likely to become aware of prostatic disorders, among men aged sixty the proportion affected by some form of disorder, no matter how mild, rises to 60 percent. At the biblical level of three score and ten it is up to 70 percent. Among those who live appreciably longer the rate accelerates until at age eighty-five and over, about 95 percent have some disorder. In many cases the disorder is so slight that it is not detected until an autopsy is performed, following death from an accident or other cause unrelated to the prostate. In these truly aged prostates, some cancer-type cells are almost always found—although the person may never have experienced any noteworthy prostatic discomfort, and certainly did not develop overt cancer.

At present there are no vaccines or other preventives against prostatic disorders. One thing that will go far to minimize their effects, however, is the awareness by every mature man that he is "at risk," and that his chances of avoiding serious difficulties depend upon his acknowledgment of this fact and his readiness to seek medical help. In addition to a general checkup every year or oftener, he should be prepared to see a doctor at the first sign of pain or discomfort.

Fortunately, an impressive majority of prostatic troubles are not life-threatening. But virtually all can subject their victims to nagging discomfort or severe pain, as well as inconvenience and embarrassment. Physicians and other health professionals justifiably put great emphasis on measures to promote early detection of cancer, but constant vigilance is equally desirable for the recognition of other prostatic disorders, however benign. If they are neglected, they are likely to cause increasing misery and also to become resistant to therapy, while prompt diagnosis and treatment will generally alleviate or cure them.

No layman can expect to diagnose—let alone treat —a prostate disorder, but everyone can learn to recognize the symptoms of probable prostatic disorders so as to seek medical advice and treatment when needed. Until recent years remarkably few men have had even an elementary knowledge of the prostate and its problems. Although this organ is essential to sexual functions, it is not visible like the external genitalia but is hidden inside the body. And being associated with both sex activities and urination, the prostate fell under the Victorian taboo of subjects not discussed in public and certainly not in mixed company. At a stag dinner a man might report his treatment for prostate trouble and his prurient drinking companions would immediately ask him about the effects on his sex life. Rectal examination of the prostate by a doctor's gloved finger was a common subject of sophomoric attempts at humor. And that was usually the extent of the attention paid to the prostate by laymen.

Times have changed, and for the better. Fewer and fewer men feel embarrassment in discussing their concealed gland, even in the presence of women, and increasing numbers are seeking regular physical checkups in which the prostate is palpated. So far, so good. But these changes in attitude and behavior have not gone far enough. Many more men need to be aware that a burning sensation in the urethra around the time of urination or after ejaculation at orgasm may be a valuable early warning of a prostatic disorder that can be cured if treated promptly. (It can also result from an infection of the kidneys or bladder, which also demands medical care.) It should not be laughed off as just a "cold on the kidneys" or in the bladder, for these organs are not susceptible to "colds": infections, yes; colds, no.

Other early symptoms are also useful as warnings: difficulty in starting to urinate; an unsteady, weak stream that fails to empty the bladder; sudden, urgent need to urinate when the nearest men's room may be blocks or miles away. Perhaps the commonest symptoms are simply frequency of the need to urinate, and the classic one that besets so many older men—waking in the dark of the morning to hurry to the bathroom.

None of these need or should cause panic, but neither should they be ignored. They should be treated with respect and then, after a visit to a doctor, with medication.

Wider recognition of the importance of the prostate in relation to sexual potency should not, by unfortunate irony, make men reluctant to accept definitive treatment for their disorders. Medicinal treatment for infections should obviously be expected to improve a man's sexual ability, but when surgery is recommended for the relief of recurrent prostatitis or benign hypertrophy (enlargement), some men refuse or postpone the operation because they mistakenly fear that impotence will follow. The fact is that many men are impotent from psychological causes before they need prostatic surgery; if they are impotent afterward they blame this upon the operation, suppressing the memory of their earlier handicap. Such self-deception and related problems of sexual performance before and after an operation require preoperative counseling by a sensitive, psychiatrically oriented urologist—a type that is rare but worth searching for.

This book has four objectives. One is to acquaint men of all ages with the basic facts of prostatic health and disease. The second is to encourage men to seek medical attention at the first signs of disorder. The third is to recommend routine rectal examinations at earlier ages and more frequently than is customary now. Physicians who emphasize the advantages of preventive over curative medicine or corrective surgery can make a significant contribution by emphasizing the importance of this simple procedure to patients approaching middle age. The fourth objective is to show that although the prostate is still in many ways a mystery to medical researchers as well as laymen, recent research has much improved the patient's chances of obtaining relief or a cure. And research currently in progress is certain to lead, well within the lifetime of today's readers, to still more significant advances.

Cancer is the disease that both men and women now dread most, and with good reason. If the statistics for prostatic cancer are taken out of context they appear unduly alarming: 60,000 new cases diagnosed in the United States in 1976, with 19,000 or more deaths. But against the perspective of 30 million men "at risk," the annual incidence of this disease should not cause panic. It should also be noted that of 250,000 operations performed annually in the United States for removal of all or part of the prostate, no fewer than 95 percent and perhaps as many as 99 percent are for noncancerous conditions. Cancer is, however, the subject of recently intensified medical research at the federal, state, and private levels. And this research has led to the development of improved X-ray techniques for reducing and retarding, perhaps even preventing, the spread of the disease, as well as to more potent medicinal treatments.

Some doctors have called this last quarter of the twentieth century "the age of prostatism." But the darkest days of the age are over, and the process of enlightenment should continue to accelerate.

Chapter
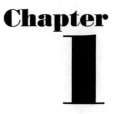

Down the Ages

The prostate is as old as mammals—at least a hundred million years. Yet the prostate was not recognized as a separate organ for more than 99 percent of those hundred million years. Nature has built into every creature a natural life span, extending from a year or two in the mouse to thirty or forty years in primitive man. It is doubtful that any man in the Stone Age lived long enough to develop prostate disease. Life expectancy in those times must have been at most twenty years, and forty would have been considered a great age indeed. It was not until man had evolved into *Homo sapiens* that he began to find means of prolonging life into those decades when the prostate begins to give trouble (roughly 50,000 years ago, although anthropologists disagree among themselves).

We can safely assume that most noninfectious prostatic disorders resulted from man's prolongation of his life expectancy. This began when he learned to use fire deliberately and purposefully to improve his skills in hunting, in preparing food, and, perhaps most important, in keeping himself from freezing to death in times of extreme cold. The use of fire, combined with the invention of improved tools, undoubtedly increased the life span—by exactly how much we do not know, but we can be fairly certain that at this time in human history a life span of forty years was not so uncommon.

This brings us into seeming conflict with the later but still ancient "three score years and ten" of the biblical period. But we must recognize that this was regarded as an extremely desirable old age for a person who had survived the hazards of childbirth, the infections of early childhood, the high incidence of accidents, the hazards of those infectious diseases that commonly afflicted young adults—notably tuberculosis—and finally the risks of death in war, on the battlefield or in capture or enslavement. If a man of King Solomon's time had survived to the age of forty he was probably immune to virtually all the diseases just mentioned and could reasonably expect to continue living for three more decades.

It would be during these last two or three decades of that seventy-year life span that he would become susceptible to disorders of the prostate, of which his priests or medicine men had no knowledge, and which they would be almost completely incompetent to diagnose or to treat.

One probable reason for the failure of the ancients to recognize the importance of the prostate is that they had discovered much earlier the most conspicuous effects of castration. They had long used castration in connection with their domestic animals, notably to convert a potentially dangerous young bull into an ox. Eventually the technique was applied to captured warriors, who were then enslaved. A result of this practice was that the effects of the prostate upon the normal aging male were obscured.

We can be certain that the medicine men of the Mesopotamian and Egyptian empires had no intellectual interest in the physiological effects of castration upon the victims' urinary systems, and they were of course entirely ignorant of the fact that the prostate is activated primarily by testosterone produced in the testicles. It is just possible, but not provable, that they made one clinical observation: a harem slave who was well fed and not overworked might outlive his masters and suffer no urinary difficulties. (Slaves used in building temples or digging canals probably did not live long enough to enjoy such a difference in survival.) And no castrated slave is likely to have developed prostate cancer.

It is one of the supreme ironies of the history of man's inhumanity to man that a great medical discovery of the mid-twentieth century, deemed worthy of a Nobel prize, was the value of castration in the control of incurable prostatic cancer. Human castration had been morally disapproved for hundreds of years, despite its being continued into the nineteenth century to provide choristers for the Vatican. It has now been restored to medicosurgical respectability, provided it is performed only for the most rigidly defined purpose, under optimal hospital conditions, and with consent. As such, it has been euphemistically renamed "bilateral orchiectomy."

If urinary disorders had developed among aging

castrated slaves as commonly as among free men or their royal masters, it is likely that they would have been dissected even while still alive, in an attempt to find the cause of the trouble. It is possible that the identity of the prostate and some clues to its functions might have been discerned. But no such procedure would have been acceptable for free men or for members of the ruling castes. The paradoxical result was that the elders of the upper classes, with their testicles intact, were prey to the deadliest of prostatic diseases, whereas their castrated slaves were not.

The ancient physicians resembled their modern counterparts in one important respect: even if they did not recognize the cause of a disorder, they were more than ready to treat its symptoms. Treatment of disorders of the prostate began even before the organ itself was clearly defined and certainly many centuries before its functions were recognized. This is roughly comparable to the work of the Inca medicine men who discovered the virtues of cinchona (or "Jesuits' bark"), which yields quinine, as a treatment for malaria many centuries before anyone learned the nature of the parasitic infection carried by mosquitoes.

The most obvious early symptom of prostate disorder is difficulty in urination. If this develops to the most severe and perceptible form, it causes a back pressure in the bladder. This elastic organ may swell to such an extent that it causes distention of the abdomen and acute distress, sometimes to the point of agonizing pain. Although it is impossible to resolve all the arguments among the various cryptographers

trying to translate ancient papyri into more understandable modern language, it seems clear that the
Egyptians of four or five thousand years ago employed remarkably modern devices to empty the
bladder and thereby relieve the pressure.

They used reeds, or copper or silver tubes, which
they inserted into the urethra to draw off the urine retained in the bladder. The resulting outflow was un-
mistakable, and in some cases there was solid evidence
of the success of the procedure. When urine is retained for a long time in the bladder, some of its
chemical contents tend to crystallize into small grav-
elly stones. These were also excreted through the
tubes (now called catheters). The medicine men seem
to have been less concerned with the volume of urine
they were removing than with the stones, and conse-
quently they became known as lithologists. Ancient
writers in several countries described swellings and
what they called "carnosities" around the neck of the
bladder. These obviously represented some form of
prostatism. The ancients did not know, however,
that by inserting a catheter into the bladder they
were passing it through the part of the urethra that
was being squeezed shut by enlargement of the prostate. What they were doing was treating the symptom with no knowledge of the cause.

It is probable that the first description of the prostate gland in any form recognizable to us was that
by Herophilus of Chalcedon, the Greek surgeon who
founded a school of anatomy in Alexandria around
300 B.C. Writings on medical as on many other matters from such early times are so fragmentary that it

is impossible to be sure what Herophilus had actually seen or was describing.

In the second century A.D. Rufus of Ephesus gave the name "parastatus glandulus" to something that may have been the prostate, but just what he meant by the term is unclear. Other ancient writers used a feminine plural form, "parastatae glandulae," which suggests that they were referring to the seminal vesicles, which are paired. The word "prostate," derives from the Latin for "standing before or beside" and was in use by the seventeenth century. Who first employed it is in dispute, and no one seems clear about what it was thought to be standing before or beside. There is no etymological relationship between "prostate" and "prostitute" or "prostrate."

It is impossible to determine how much prostatic disorder from the seventeenth century through the nineteenth was caused by simple benign hypertrophy, how much by infection—then usually the result of gonorrhea—and how much developed from causes that were and sometimes still are unknown. (In modern times the word prostatosis, meaning simply disorder of the prostate, has been used for the latter group.) There is, further, no way of ascertaining how much prostatic disease was cancerous. This is partly because of the ignorance prevailing in regard to the prostate itself, but largely because of the attitude toward cancer: until the beginning of the twentieth century cancer was considered a foul, probably contagious disease, related to sexual overindulgence, perversion, or venereal infection.

For more than four thousand years, from the time

of the Pharaonic physicians to the seventeenth century, the only conspicuous advance in the treatment of prostatic disorders—and this had no bearing upon the underlying disease—was Ambroise Paré's development of a curved tube with a retractable cutting wire passed through it. This sixteenth-century instrument, inserted through the urethra to remove excess tissue, was a direct ancestor of today's sophisticated resectoscope.

Not surprisingly, little constructive treatment of prostate disorders was possible until the anatomy and the physiological functions of the organ were better understood. This did not develop until the end of the nineteenth century, and the process is still far from complete. Surgery without undue risk of death from accidental infection became possible only with the development, in the mid-nineteenth century, of anesthesia and of Lord Lister's first antiseptic and then aseptic procedures.

When it became apparent that the prostate, in addition to being an important organ in the male's physiological processes—notably his sexual ability—was also capable of becoming the site of a malignant cancer, the idea of removing the entire organ emerged. It is still not certain when the first removal of an entire prostate (a true prostatectomy) was achieved. An Italian surgeon, Enrico Bottini, reported in Berlin in 1890 that he had performed such an operation. If other surgeons were impressed, they decided that emulation was the sincerest form of praise, and returned to their operating rooms to develop similar techniques. Controversy continues as to how radical or total the nineteenth-century operations were, and the words themselves are subject to overlapping definitions.

An amusing episode in the unending controversy over prostate surgery involves an ebullient surgeon from western Ireland, Patrick (later Sir Patrick) Freyer. He apparently claimed more credit than his due for having performed what he contended was a total extirpation of the prostate without damage to the patient's urinary or sexual functions—a surgical feat that is considered impossible even today. The vivid but imprecise reporting of his procedure resulted in an extraordinarily bitter transatlantic controversy with an American urologist who claimed to have achieved comparable effects but by slightly different methods. However, Freyer, who pronounced his name to rhyme with beer, made a sufficient contribution to the cause of prostate therapy that Lord Moynihan, the great English surgeon, is supposed to have said, "That Galway man was aptly named 'Pee-Freer.' "

As late as 1974 a veteran urologist recently retired from practice wrote, "The sole function of the prostate is to produce a lubricating fluid to transport sperm cells during sex relations." This may have been accepted as fact during that elderly physician's time in medical school, forty or more years earlier, but so simple a concept of the prostate has been virtually wiped out in the years of medical research since then.

Dr. Charles B. Huggins, winner of a Nobel prize for his great contribution to the treatment, both medical and surgical, of prostatic cancer, has compared the modern medical scientist's knowledge of the prostate with the impressions of the six blind men who examined an elephant and each described a different characteristic. Dr. Huggins believes that science knows little more about the biology of prostatic cells than the blind men knew of the elephant's anatomy.

Dr. Gerald P. Murphy, Director of the National Prostatic Cancer Project of the National Institutes of Health, says the prostate is "an organ of mystery" even now. Dr. Aaron Bendich, of the Sloan-Kettering Institute for Cancer Research, goes further and insists that investigators have not begun to understand even superficially the exquisitely delicate biological—meaning primarily biochemical—functions that arise from the anatomy of the prostate.

What *is* certain today is that the prostate is an enormously complex chemical factory, producing both enzymes and hormones. The history of the prostate is now being written and rewritten in the laboratories of investigators who are, both literally and figuratively, taking a new look at the gland, using exquisitely refined techniques unknown to their forebears.

Chapter 2

Anatomy

Although we know the ancients lacked the delicate surgical instruments of today, their slowness in recognizing even the existence of the prostate is almost incomprehensible. The lack of research during the Dark Ages and Middle Ages is more understandable, because at that time dissection of the human corpse was discouraged or flatly forbidden in most cultures, primarily for religious reasons.

It remained for Vesalius, who lived from 1514 to 1565, to defy the edicts of the Church and rob the crows and vultures of the corpses of executed men so that he could dissect them with his somewhat primitive scalpel. In his anatomical masterpieces, published in 1538 and 1543, he showed what can be recognized with fair certainty as the prostate. However, there is an anomaly even in this work by a great master. The shape of the gland as he shows it is more like that of the dog than the human.

In the newborn "man child," the prostate may be hardly bigger than a grain of barley, but a physician's examining finger can feel it in the wall of the rectum. It develops during gestation under the influence of the mother's hormones, which are not exclusively estrogenic (female types) but partly androgenic (male types). During infancy the prostate remains static and therefore appears to decrease in relative size. It does not resume growth until puberty, when the testicles begin to produce the testosterone that causes the prostate to grow to its adult size. At the end of adolescence, about the age of eighteen, the master pituitary gland gives the signal for the growth hormone (somatotropin) to halt its promotion of growth in general. The growth of the prostate also stops at this time, not because of a decrease in its supply of testosterone but because this masculine hormone has another function, which now takes precedence: to stimulate the production of sperm.

Since men vary so much in overall size, there is also considerable variation in the size of their internal organs. Anatomists figure that the average, normal adult man has a prostate gland which measures 30 mm. to 40 mm. vertically, and we can translate this roughly (since all the figures are approximations) into $1\frac{1}{4}$ in. to $1\frac{3}{4}$ in. Its largest dimension is horizontal, 40 mm. or $1\frac{3}{4}$ in., or perhaps 50 mm. or 2 in. The smallest dimension is its thickness, which averages only about 20 mm. or 4/5 in. A healthy man's normal prostate weighs 20 grams or a little more—less than $\frac{3}{4}$ oz.

Although we usually think of the prostate as a "gland," this is not completely accurate. A gland is a combination of cells that secrete (manufacture) biochemical substances important to the function of the human system. The prostate is not a single gland

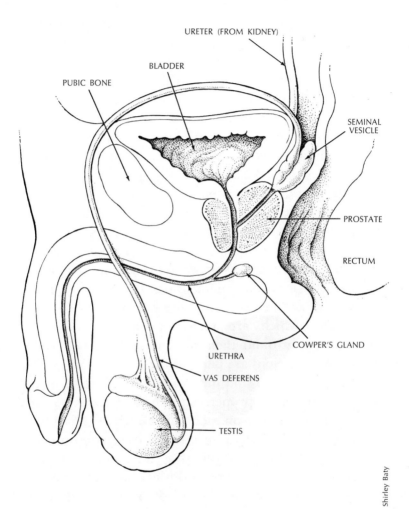

URETER (FROM KIDNEY)

BLADDER

PUBIC BONE

SEMINAL
VESICLE

PROSTATE

RECTUM

COWPER'S GLAND

URETHRA

VAS DEFERENS

TESTIS

Shirley Baty

THE UROGENITAL SYSTEM

but an accumulation of several glandular, secreting parts interwoven with fibrous and muscular structures. No less an authority than Dr. William Wallace Scott, of Johns Hopkins Hospital, says that there is still considerable controversy about the origin and development of the human prostate, and especially about its division into lobes—some physiologists call them areas or zones—and the functions that each performs. Anatomists' opinions about the number of glandular parts vary from three to seven, but when the specialists describe the prostate's structure in detail, most of them enumerate five lobes.

In addition to these lobes the prostate contains a number of other structures which have important effects upon urinary function and sexual activity. Since the prostate surrounds the beginning of the urethra, it is convenient to describe it from the inside out. Closest to the urethra are the mucosal glands, which are relatively short and simple. Wrapped around them are the submucosal glands, whose functions are perhaps the least obvious of all, while the third and outermost band consists of the prostatic glands proper. These have long ducts which enter the urethra on each side. One body of opinion holds that the true prostatic glands are separated by a definite fibrous capsule from the mucosal and submucosal glands. But even this distinction is not universally accepted, for in a study of two hundred autopsy specimens this postulated capsule could not always be found.

A widely accepted description of the anatomy of the prostate, based on the five-lobe concept, counts

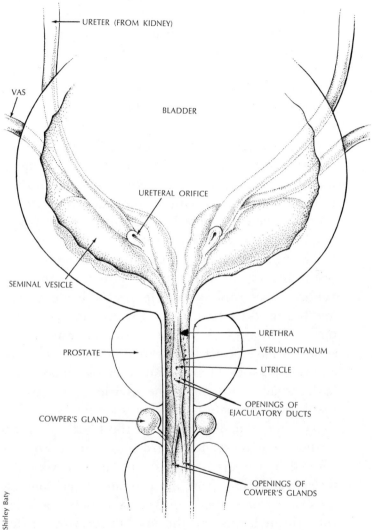

URETER (FROM KIDNEY)

VAS

BLADDER

URETERAL ORIFICE

SEMINAL VESICLE

PROSTATE

COWPER'S GLAND

URETHRA

VERUMONTANUM

UTRICLE

OPENINGS OF
EJACULATORY DUCTS

OPENINGS OF
COWPER'S GLANDS

Shirley Baty

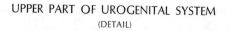

UPPER PART OF UROGENITAL SYSTEM
(DETAIL)

first the posterior—meaning that it projects slightly backward into the rectum; this is the part that can be felt by the gloved finger of the examining physician. Then there is a middle lobe of uncertain function, and there are two lateral lobes, one on each side, while forward (toward the abdominal cavity) is an anterior lobe. The posterior lobe, the one that is palpable in the rectum, is the one least likely to be involved in common urinary difficulties, unless it becomes cancerous. It is more susceptible to cancer than the other lobes. The median, lateral, and anterior lobes are most subject to overgrowth without cancer, a condition known as benign prostatic hypertrophy, or BPH (see Chapter Seven).

The prostate is directly beneath the bladder, at the beginning of the urethra, the outlet channel for voiding. When the urethra leaves the bladder neck and begins its course through the prostate it encounters a minor obstacle, the verumontanum. This seems to have no particular anatomical significance and is like a little bump on an otherwise smooth surface. Adjacent to this is the utricle genicularis, a small piece of male tissue corresponding in evolutionary terms to the uterus in the female. A little farther along on its downward course, the urethra is entered by the ejaculatory ducts, through which it receives secretions from the prostate. Then comes a little narrowing called the urethral crest. After it has gone through this gap the urethra receives further injections of secretions from Cowper's glands. Beyond this point and still proceeding downward, the urethra becomes a more simple line carrying urine

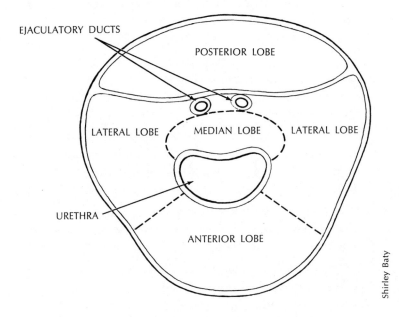

EJACULATORY DUCTS

POSTERIOR LOBE

LATERAL LOBE MEDIAN LOBE LATERAL LOBE

URETHRA

ANTERIOR LOBE

Shirley Baty

HORIZONTAL CROSS-SECTION
OF A NORMAL PROSTATE

or semen. Many women complain that in devising the human reproductive system nature was extraordinarily inconsiderate of the female, subjecting her to decades of periodic discomfort as well as the burdens of pregnancy and lactation. Only the most chauvinistic male could disagree, but the same male might contend that in designing his genitourinary system nature ignored all rules of sensible design and made him prey to a variety of disorders. First, it defied the maxim that a straight line is the shortest distance between two points, and devised instead a labyrinthine machinery for insemination. In a man of normal proportions the distance between the testicles where the spermatozoa are manufactured and the penis through which they will be ejected is not more than 5 centimeters, or about 2 inches. However, in nature's plan the distance is four or five times as great and many complex biochemical processes take place along this route.

Since the Latin plurals of some of these anatomical words are cumbersome, it is easiest if we simply take the functioning of one testicle and its product. The spermatozoa are manufactured in the testicles. From there several small tubes deliver the sperm into the vas deferens—Latin for "carrying-away vessel." The sperm, which resemble miniature tadpoles, number in the millions. However, they need energy and nourishment to equip them completely for the final task of fertilization. Each vas deferens, one on each side for each testicle, winds past a bend in the penis, beyond the pubic bone, and up to the level of the bladder, before it turns and enters the prostate. Almost exactly coinciding with this point of entry is a pair of small organs called the seminal vesicles, which produce fructose (milk sugar) to give the sperm the quick energy they need for their continued journey. No other human organ produces this sugar. After the sperm have been vitalized in this way and are en route to their destination they still must receive secretions from the prostatic ducts, to supply a sufficient volume of fluid for ease of flow. And after the urethra is past the prostate there is a further injection of material from Cowper's glands.

When the penis becomes erect, the sphincter at the lower end of the bladder, where the urethra begins its passage through the prostate, closes so that urine cannot mix with the seminal ejaculate. There is a second sphincter farther down which also closes as double insurance. Except for a few instances that may begin with congenital defects or a childhood illness, it is usual for a man to approach the age of fifty without having urinary difficulty resulting from a disorder of the sphincters. Some nervous conditions may impair control of voiding, but in later life most such problems originate in the prostate itself.

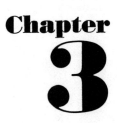

Chapter 3

Symptoms, Signs, and Nonsymptoms

In prostatic disorders, as in other human illnesses, the symptoms may be similar for different conditions. These symptoms, already noted briefly, are frequent, urgent, and painful or difficult urination. The need to get up in the middle of the night to urinate is principally associated with advancing age and a loss of muscle tone in the sphincters. Other symptoms, such as fever and pain in the joints, are usually indications of more specific complaints and will be discussed in chapters dealing with these.

Since there are certain urinary disorders to which the human male is liable from birth, but which have nothing to do with the chronological development of the adult prostate, we may discuss these first. As a result of either genetically determined defects, or factors operating during pregnancy, it is possible for a baby to be born with abnormalities of the urinary tract. These are matters for the pediatric urologist. Somewhat less frequently an adolescent or young adult will have urinary problems which again are not associated with the developing prostate gland itself.

There are also adult conditions that have nothing to do with prostatic disease but that may nevertheless confuse the health-conscious layman. While there is some difference of opinion as to the relative holding capacity or elasticity of the female and male bladders, there is no question that changes in weather often produce temporary changes in urinary performance. If a resident of northern latitudes takes a two-week winter vacation in the sunny south, he or she is almost certain to spend a good deal of time playing tennis or sunbathing. In either case there will be a considerable dispersal of body water through the sweat glands. This phenomenon was verified back in the eighteenth century, in the somewhat unpromising climate of England, by the scientist John Dalton, who carefully weighed his intake of solid and liquid matter, and thereafter with equal care weighed the amount of solid and liquid matter he excreted. He found that there was a marked discrepancy between his liquid intake and his measurable liquid output because of the amount of liquid he lost through perspiration and through the moist air he exhaled while breathing.

If a vacationer returns from the south to go skiing in the north, he or she immediately covers the body with layer upon layer of clothing, and most of these layers are impervious to moisture. As a result, very little moisture is lost through the sweat glands. The effect is that a person of either sex who normally urinates every two, three, or four hours suddenly finds himself needing to do so at intervals of an hour or so, and often with a sense of considerable urgency.

This, it must be emphasized, is an effect of climatic conditions upon the body's physiological processes, complicated by the amount of clothing that is worn, and it has nothing to do with the health of the urinary tract.

A more familiar example of change in frequency involves a man who has a breakfast of orange juice and two cups of coffee and rushes off to work. While walking at his customary pace to his office, but in unaccustomedly cold weather, he suddenly feels an urgent need for a men's room. In most of our cities nowadays, largely as a result of security procedures, it is often difficult for him to find one. He has the option of either confronting a security guard in an unfamiliar building, and asking directions to the men's room and permission to use it, or of simply gritting his teeth and going on to his own office where the facilities are immediately available. Urologists have issued a stern warning—to women as well as men— that it is inadvisable to postpone urination except when absolutely necessary, as doing so increases the risk of bladder and kidney infections. On city streets, superhighways, and in unfamiliar territory anywhere, we have a difficult choice between possible embarrassment and defying medical opinion.

It is generally known that both caffeine and alcohol act as diuretics—that is, they increase the tendency for the kidneys to process urine out of the bloodstream and pour it through the ureters into the bladder. This explains why, after lavish business lunches, preceded by two or more cocktails and followed by coffee, many men must immediately go to the washroom. The severity of the effects of caffeine and alcohol varies from person to person. However severe it may be, it is most unlikely to constitute a symptom of sufficient importance to justify a visit to a doctor.

There is a widespread belief that an urgent need to urinate, or pain in the urethra immediately following urination, may be caused by either excessive sexual activity or absence of sexual activity, or, especially in the older adolescent approaching maturity, by masturbation. Some of these old, moralistic doctors' tales should obviously be dismissed. Reliable case histories of many patients do, however, indicate that an abrupt or extreme change in sexual activity—either an increase or a decrease—may produce at least temporary prostatic symptoms.

One of the reasons for mistaken beliefs about the human prostate is the equally mistaken belief that the human species is virtually the only one capable of sexual activity and reproduction day in and day out, throughout the year. This is based upon the common knowledge that among many animals, especially domesticated species, sexual activity is absent or minimal except when the male is excited by the odor of a female in heat. The fact is that many species of animals, not only primates but those of the so-called lower orders, are capable of sexual responses and activities virtually throughout the year, without the necessity for the male's being stimulated by a female in heat.

Our general conclusion must be that the males of most of the higher animals continuously secrete spermatozoa, that they continuously move these spermatozoa through a complex system to a point at which they are capable of ejaculation at any time following some form of sexual stimulation. If there is no such climactic event as ejaculation, the prostatic secretions, carrying other secretions with them, and, most important, carrying old, infertile spermatozoa, trickle into the urethra. From this they are expelled during normal urination without any awareness of this process by the man or monkey concerned.

There is one other kind of urinary difficulty that should be eliminated from the group associated with the prostate. Any inflammation of any part of the urinary tract from the kidneys to the outlet of the urethra is almost certain to produce discomfort— most commonly a burning sensation upon urination. If the inflammation occurs in the kidneys it is technically nephritis, although that is a word that most urologists prefer to avoid because they tend to reserve it for a more serious disease. It can usually be treated with antimicrobial drugs and need not lead to any persistent difficulties. A little farther down the urinary tract, the bladder is even more susceptible to infection, and this form of disorder is called cystitis. Although it may be caused by a wide variety of infectious agents, cystitis does not commonly yield to treatment by antibiotics. As a result, the drugs preferred for treatment are the sulfas. If the urethra itself becomes inflamed as a result of an infection, the preferred drugs for treatment in this area are also the sulfas.

Chapter

Infectious Prostatitis

Although infections of the prostate are relatively rare among young men, they are the most common types of disease affecting this gland in the middle decades of life. They occur in two major forms, called acute and chronic, and it must be emphasized that these words convey no information about the severity of the disorder but refer only to abruptness of onset and probable duration. The acute comes on more suddenly and is not likely to last long, whereas the chronic may persist for years, with intermissions of freedom from distress punctuated by relapses. Either kind of infectious prostatitis may result from invasion by one or more of several distinct species of microbes. When a man arrives at a urologist's office with distressing complaints suggesting severe prostatitis, even the most expert diagnostician sometimes faces difficult challenges. The patient needs to be prepared for this: he cannot expect instant, simple answers to highly complex questions.

In some cases a prostatic infection is detected before the patient has become aware of any symptoms. This may occur if a man has had a routine physical checkup and been given what appears to be a clean bill of health—until the laboratory report shows the presence of pus cells, blood cells, or bacterial debris in his urine. Such a finding should send the man to a urologist, who will then conduct further tests to ascertain the site and nature of the infection.

Far more typical is the man who has some or all of the common urinary difficulties already listed, and perhaps others more distressing so that he cannot ignore his distress.

The diagnosing physician first needs a detailed and accurate history of the patient's genitourinary symptoms. If these have developed suddenly, both doctor and patient may be fortunate: the disorder may be a true first attack of acute infectious prostatitis, and effective treatment is usually straightforward.

Delay in reporting symptoms is a source of frustration and confusion for the urologist. When asked how long they have been bothering him, a patient may reply that he first noticed discomfort several months or a year ago, but figured that he could live with it. Or perhaps he thought it was an aspect of the normal process of aging. The urologist must be forgiven if he shows some irritation as he says, "If you'd come to me six months ago, you almost certainly wouldn't be in this trouble now."

When the doctor believes he is confronted with a case of infectious prostatitis, he must try hard to find out whether this is indeed a first attack. Some patients are genuinely unable to give a reliable answer, for often the first episode is so mild that they do not suspect prostatic disease. Getting an accurate case history is further complicated by the fact that many men are reluctant to disclose details of their sex life, especially to a doctor they are consulting for the first time. This is a serious mistake, because some prostatic infections are clearly associated with sexual practices. The more the doctor knows about the probable origin of an infection, the better his chances of curing it.

The patient who lies about his earlier troubles is even more baffling to the urologist. A man may have been effectively treated for his first bout of acute prostatitis, and apparently cured, only to have the infection flare up again within a few weeks or months. After two or three such episodes this patient is likely to seek help from another doctor in the hope of obtaining permanent relief through the magic of some more potent medication. Disappointed again, he continues "doctor shopping." Such a patient's distress is understandable, but there is less reason now than in former years for his behavior. Although the sulfas and antibiotics have long since established their value against acute infections, until recently no medicine could be relied upon for long-lasting suppression of chronic conditions. There is now a medication that holds great promise of achieving this result for many patients. How it may be prescribed is still unclear until government regulations are clarified. This is a combination drug with a ten-syllable name, usually called by its initials, TMP-SMZ.

When a man consults a urologist complaining of both the standard urinary difficulties and additional symptoms such as alternating chills and feverish episodes, pain in the lower back or the perineal area (between anus and scrotum), or aching joints and muscles, the chances are that he has acute infectious prostatitis. But for a confirming diagnosis both a physical examination and laboratory tests are necessary. If the physician finds that there is tenderness when he exerts gentle pressure on different parts of the lower abdomen and pelvis, this may tell him something significant about swollen organs. An important and familiar feature of this examination is almost as simple—the insertion of a gloved finger into the rectum, to palpate the rear wall of the prostate. The physician is as concerned as the patient to make sure that he is not dealing with a case of cancer. If he does not feel hard, irregular lumps in the prostate he can be fairly confident in ruling out cancer. If he feels smooth, regular lumps they are most likely calcified stones (calculi) like those commonly found in other parts of the body. As these are benign they can usually be ignored.

Other tests involve collecting specimens of urine and prostatic fluid and developing cultures from them in the laboratory to see which bacteria grow. At different times and different medical centers urologists have used a number of variations of this basic technique. The one now regarded as the most informative was developed and refined at Stanford University Medical Center. The previous methods had been generally considered adequate for diagnosing acute infections but had been unsatisfactory in relation to the chronic forms.

In 1965 a team of urological investigators at Stanford, headed by Dr. Thomas A. Stamey and Dr. Edwin M. Meares, Jr., devised what they first thought was a nearly foolproof technique for determining whether a patient had infectious prostatitis and what kind of bacteria caused it. In its original form the procedure consisted of taking three specimens of urine from the patient at short intervals, the first at the beginning of urination, the second after a considerable volume of urine had been voided and discarded, and the third after the prostate had been gently massaged. (The massage must be done with very light pressure, as otherwise an acute infection might be aggravated.) Dr. Stamey soon conceded: "From these studies we mistakenly concluded that chronic bacterial prostatitis was not a common disease." Such a conclusion seemed so at variance with hospital experience that the investigators continued their work, modified the technique, and now use a process that requires the collection of four specimens. This method establishes, with a high degree of accuracy, whether the patient is suffering from infectious prostatitis. The question whether it is of the chronic type may take longer to resolve.

The patient is required to drink a sufficient quantity of fluid to insure that he will arrive for the examination with a full bladder. Then when he begins to urinate, the first 10 c.c.s. (about one third of a fluid ounce) are collected. This portion is designated VB-1, for Void Bladder No. 1. Next, a considerable quantity of urine is excreted until the patient is reasonably comfortable, and this part is discarded. Before further urination becomes impossible, a second or "midstream" sample is collected, VB-2. Third, the examining physician massages the prostate and squeezes from the prostatic ducts a small quantity of their secretions, which dribble through the urethra and are collected. Whether these few drops contain sperm or other components of seminal fluid is immaterial. Finally, a further urine sample, VB-3, is collected. All these samples are then subjected to microbial culture techniques in the laboratory.

This four-step procedure usually makes it possible for the physician to differentiate between urethral and prostatic infections. However, he cannot direct a pinpointed attack against the cause of the infection until he receives the test results. Meantime he will probably prescribe supportive measures: bed rest, fever-reducing and pain-relieving medicines such as aspirin or acetaminophen, a gentle stool softener (not a strong laxative), and a lot of fluids. Plus two prohibitions: no alcohol and no highly-spiced foods.

One diagnostic procedure which the layman is likely to have heard of and to regard with undue fear is catheterization, the insertion of a tube through the urethra to drain off excess urine retained in the bladder. This technique is not used if the urologist believes he is dealing with an acute bacterial infection because it might spread the disease. In such a case, if the bladder is so distended that it must be drained, the preferred method now is for the surgeon (using a local anesthetic) to drain the bladder through the abdominal wall. This may cause some discomfort for a day or two, but the discomfort is less than that caused by urine retention.

The layman-patient will doubtless ask his doctor how it is possible for infecting microbes to get into the prostate. The urologist will explain that the prostate is encased in a fairly impermeable capsule and is normally protected against germs in fecal matter passing down the large bowel. The prostate receives little fluid from external sources except, of course, its necessary blood supply. And because the flow of prostatic secretions is outward and downward, microbes must swim upstream against the current. Yet the nature of many prostatic infections indicates that a surprising number of them succeed in doing so. Perhaps still more surprising, colon bacilli are by far the most common cause of acute infectious prostatitis.

Dr. Meares—who is now the head of the departments of urology at Tufts University School of Medicine and the New England Medical Center Hospitals—remarks that in many cases the urologist is as puzzled as the layman about the likeliest route of infection. But it is important to find out, so that the physician can decide upon the most promising treatment and counsel his patient regarding measures that will help to ward off a recurrence. Dr. Meares lists four possible routes of infection: 1) through the blood stream; 2) from the rectum, either directly or through the lymphatic system; 3) a back flow of infected urine into the prostatic ducts; and 4) an infection ascending from the penis along the urethra. The first three are beyond the patient's ability to influence but the fourth is within his control. Gonorrheal infections of the prostate are almost invariably the result of intercourse with an infected partner, since the blood stream route of infection by gonococci is extremely rare. Similarly, infections from other organisms in the vulva and vagina can be traced directly to intercourse.

No matter what route the infecting microbes travel, once they succeed in entering the prostate they find there an ideal, temperature-controlled climate and suitable nourishment. Moreover, they are in an essentially privileged sanctuary, because most germ-killing drugs have greater difficulty in penetrating the prostate than do the germs themselves.

Gonorrhea was for centuries the prevalent cause of severe infections of the male urogenital tract, and until the middle of this century it remained extremely difficult to treat. In the early days of the antibiotic era came penicillin, and it was discovered that one or two massive injections of penicillin would cure gonorrhea almost overnight. The incidence of the disease, including infections of the prostate, declined dramatically for almost two decades. When some varieties of the gonococcus became resistant to ordinary penicillin, more potent forms of the antibiotic proved to be still effective. With the revolution in sexual mores that developed in the 1960s, gonorrhea has regained some of its former prevalence, with a resultant increase in gonococcal prostatitis. It is still true that improved forms of penicillin and some other antibiotics will effect cures so nearly instantaneous that they appear magical, but it is equally true that a cured patient can suffer a recurrence within a day or two upon intimate contact with an infected partner.

Despite the current upsurge of gonorrhea, the great majority of cases of infectious prostatitis are caused by nonvenereal microbes, and about 80 percent of the acute form are caused by *Escherichia coli*, the colon bacilli. These bacilli are normally found in the lower bowel and its fecal content. Through defective sewerage systems they can contaminate a water supply and, of course, swimming pools and bathing beaches. Usually with no warning, colon bacilli occasionally reach the lungs or bloodstream to cause pneumonia or septicemia; more commonly they infect the bladder and kidneys as well as the prostate. One obvious route of possible transmission is through careless toilet habits and some sexual practices, but such explanations do not always apply. People who are fastidious about personal hygiene may also become infected.

If the laboratory tests indicate infection with *E. coli*, the urologist is almost certain to prescribe an antibiotic for a short course of intensive treatment. Since there are many varieties of *E. coli*, there is no one antibiotic appropriate for all cases. If the lab results are not precise enough to suggest the choice of medication, the physician can perform a fairly rapid and simple screening in the test tube, to determine which antibiotic is most likely to be quickly effective. His choice will lie between the familiar penicillin-G and several recent modifications of the basic peni-

cillin (a current favorite is ampicillin), three tetra-
cyclines, and two or three other antimicrobials. Some
of these are most effective when taken by mouth;
others are injected. The choice of drug and method
of administration depend upon the doctors' judg-
ments, and there are legitimate differences of opinion among them as to which is best for any particular
patient.

One patient treated at Stanford in 1962, when he
was forty-nine years old, had such a rampaging prostatitis that his post-massage urine specimen yielded
some 187,000 colon bacilli per c.c. While he was under observation the infection ascended to his bladder. A course of oxytetracycline brought his fever
down within twenty-four hours, and in fourteen days
his prostatitis could be considered cured. During the
following three years he had three relatively minor
infections of the bladder and urethra but his prostate
was not involved. This gland remained disease-free
during many years of follow-up study.

A surprising and favorable aspect of acute infections of the prostate is that the inflammatory process
appears to facilitate the penetration of antimicrobial
drugs that are normally reluctant to pierce the gland's
protective capsule. Presumably this is because of an
increased blood supply resulting from the inflammation. Whatever the explanation, it provides valuable
assistance in treatment.

When the patient returning for a checkup (usually
within a few days or at most two weeks) appears to be
free of symptoms and gives urine specimens that are
devoid of infecting bacteria, the doctor is justified in

congratulating both the patient and himself. But he should not claim a cure, because many patients have a recurrence of their complaint within a few months, weeks, or even days. These cases fall into the general category of chronic prostatitis, to be discussed in detail later.

When infection with colon bacilli is not the principal source of a case of acute prostatitis, the cause may be one or more of a dozen other microbes. These are responsible for slightly more than 20 percent of cases because sometimes they coexist with *E. coli* in a dual infection. Most of these have forbidding Latin names, though one exception is the "blue-pus organism" that also thrives in infected wounds. Laboratory findings should indicate which, if any, of these microbes are to blame for the patient's disease, and for all of them there are antibiotics that should effect prompt cures.

For some mixed infections, caused by strains of colon bacteria and other microbes that are resistant to the most familiar antibiotics, there is another oral medication, cephaloglycin (trade name: Kafocin). And for more resistant cases there are two potent antimicrobials that are injected: gentamicin (Garamycin) and a relative of cephaloglycin, Keflin.

Urologists are far from unanimous as to how long a patient should be kept on medication, especially if the acute symptoms seem to subside quickly. To make assurance doubly sure, Dr. Meares prefers to have his patients on medication for thirty days.

All the organisms discussed so far are what microbiologists classify as bacteria. Two others have recently been found in an increasing proportion of urethral, bladder, and prostatic infections. Since both are commonly found in the vulva and vagina, they are transmitted through sexual intercourse and are technically venereal disorders, although physicians call them "nonspecific," to distinguish them from syphilis and gonorrhea. One of these organisms is a fungus, *Monilia* (or *Candida*) *albicans,* and produces the infection known as moniliasis. The second is a protozoan, a tiny form of animal life, called *Trichomonas vaginalis.* Just how often either of these organisms reaches the prostate to cause acute infection is unclear, partly because they are often involved in simultaneous bacterial infection.

When a man contracts moniliasis from an infected vulva or vagina he is likely to develop skin eruptions on the glans penis. These can be treated effectively with the antibiotic nystatin (trade name: Mycostatin) in a cream or ointment. If the monilia travel upward internally and cause urethritis the same antibiotic, taken in an oral form, is usually curative. If the fungi succeed in reaching the prostate, an inflammatory infection there is more resistant to treatment. Oral Mycostatin may be moderately effective. What is needed is an antifungal medication with greater ability to penetrate the prostate.

Trichomonas organisms can reach far up the urethra and infect the bladder, and in some cases the prostate also. A brief and effective treatment for "trich" infections is a drug called metronidazole (trade name: Flagyl). Like many such medications it may cause some gastric distress, but this is not usually severe. It is prescribed for both men and women, and because of the interchange of infectious microbes during intercourse, the wisest physicians always prescribe the drug for both partners at the same time. (For women there is a vaginal suppository form.) The idea, of course, is to knock out the infection in the partners simultaneously, otherwise either can reinfect the other almost immediately, in what is known as the "ping-pong effect." Sexual partners will be well advised to take the medication faithfully for as long as prescribed, which may be from ten days to three weeks.

Virtually all of the many microbes capable of causing acute infectious prostatitis may appear to have been eliminated by intensive treatment as previously described, and yet return to subject the patient to a renewed attack. This form of the disease is commonly called chronic, but recurrent is more descriptive. The patient almost invariably enjoys remissions of weeks or months during which he hopes and believes that he has been cured, only to be disillusioned when the familiar symptoms reappear. It is usually not clear whether the recurrence of active disease results from a few of the original infecting bacteria having remained dormant for a while and then resumed active multiplication or from reinfection by microbes to which the patient is especially susceptible. Whatever the mechanism, the effect is the same.

When the victim of chronic or recurrent prostatitis visits the urologist, he may appear less physically ill than the patient with an acute attack. Although most of the discomforting symptoms are the same, the chills and fever so characteristic of the acute attack are less likely to beset the chronic sufferer, except perhaps during unpredictable flare-ups. But emotionally he may be more disturbed, with a hopeless "Here we go again" feeling.

Until recently his despair was shared by most urologists. Their attitude was based upon a chemical technicality. Most microbe-killing drugs, both sulfas and antibiotics, are either too acidic or so insoluble in blood lipids (fats) that their potency is largely destroyed before they can enter the prostate. Despite their current success in overcoming this difficulty with appropriate medications in treating acute infections, medical investigators do not know why similar and perhaps more prolonged treatment fails in many cases of the recurrent form. For the patient suffering from a relapse, additional laboratory tests and perhaps an educated guess by the physician often lead to the prescribing of a different medication, which again alleviates the symptoms but does not prevent recurrence. Only a drug that is new to the treatment of prostatic disease in the United States, trimethoprim-sulfamethoxazole (TMP-SMZ), offers substantial new hope for curing chronic prostatitis. This medication is so remarkable in its reported effects, and so entangled in federal regulations, that it deserves a chapter to itself.

Until about 1973, when the potency of TMP-SMZ began to be demonstrated, it was widely believed that the only cure for chronic or recurrent prostatitis lay in surgery. Although surgical intervention is emphatically not to be considered for acute infectious prostatitis (as it might spread the infection), some urologists held that it was possible to cut out parts of the gland that might harbor dormant bacteria or be susceptible to reinfection. The procedure used was the transurethral resection (TUR), in which the modern electrical equivalents of Ambroise Paré's fine cutting tools are inserted through the urethra. What proportion of chronic sufferers have been cured by this operation is unknown—a cured patient may not return to his doctor to report, whereas one who is not cured will continue doctor shopping. A far more drastic operation, total prostatectomy (removal of the entire gland) has sometimes been performed for chronic prostatitis. But most patients, except perhaps the most aged, refuse to undergo this as it is virtually certain to result in impotence, whereas a TUR need have no such sequel.

Chapter
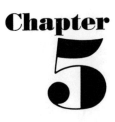

The More Wondrous Drug

When patients with a chronic and possibly incurable disease make the rounds from one doctor's office or medical center to another, hoping to get a prescription for a more wonderful drug than the last one they took, physicians are understandably irritated. They feel that this reflects unfairly upon their own skills. This is not so in regard to chronic infectious prostatitis.

Many of the most eminent American and a still greater proportion of European specialists in the treatment of infectious diseases believe that—for once—the patient is right and that the more wondrous drug actually exists. But for years the regulatory routines of the United States Food and Drug Administration have held up its approval for general use by urologists and other physicians for the treatment of bacterial prostatitis. This is more puzzling than most bureaucratic confusional states, because the drug was approved early in 1974 as a generally available medication for the treatment of urinary tract infections, including those suffered by women (subject to the usual warning about taking any drug during pregnancy). For these conditions it has long been widely advertised (to doctors only) by two large and reputable international pharmaceutical companies: Burroughs Wellcome Co., which calls its brand Septra, and Roche Laboratories, using the name Bactrim for the identical product. This medication is actually a combination of two drugs, trimethoprim (80 mg., or one part) and sulfamethoxazole (400 mg., or five parts)—or TMP-SMZ as a short handle. Trimethoprim has not been approved in the United States for use alone.

Trimethoprim is of particular interest because it is virtually the first, if not actually the first, antibacterial synthesized on the basis of logical deductions from knowledge of the metabolic processes of bacteria. This is in sharp contrast to the historical pattern in which almost every useful drug, from willow-bark tea (aspirin) and cinchona to the sulfas and antibiotics, has had its usefulness explained only long after it had been discovered by trial and error.

The synthesis of trimethoprim grew out of the discovery in the 1940s of drugs that interfere selectively with the metabolism of cancer cells. One-celled bacteria need folic acid (or a close chemical relative) just as individual human cells do, but they cannot produce it by the same metabolic pathways. So Dr. George H. Hitchings of Burroughs Wellcome set out to find a substance that would block the metabolic pathway in the bacterial cell but not in the human cell. He and his colleagues found it in trimethoprim. Some of the sulfas have a similar blocking effect at a different stage in the bacterial metabolic chain, but they do not readily penetrate the sanctuary of the prostate. What emerged from this research was an antimicrobial combination that operates on the old "one-two" principle: let the sulfa do its best against infecting bacteria, then let trimethoprim, which enters the prostate more easily and in greater proportion than any other medication so far known, take over for the kill.

The combination was approved in Britain (where it is called cotrimoxazole) and by 1968 was in wide use there for conditions as diverse as upper respiratory and urinary tract infections, including gonorrhea. When the U.S. Food and Drug Administration gave its limited, belated approval six years later, the *Journal of the American Medical Association* ran an editorial with the unaccustomedly sardonic title "Better Late than Never." But that F.D.A. approval extended only to "urinary tract" infections, and by F.D.A. definition the prostate is a part not of the urinary tract but of the genital system. The responsible officials in the F.D.A. are aware of the interrelationship of the urogenital tract and the prostate, but remain unmoved by the fact that the most distinguished urologists regard—and *treat*—the two as inseparable. Considering the intimate physical contact and the biochemical interchanges between the urinary and prostatic systems, the F.D.A.'s refusal to consider them together can only be regarded as an outmoded psychological hang-up.

Another F.D.A. hang-up involves medicines in fixed combinations. There is a valid rationale for this, but only up to a point. In the 1950s and early

1960s some pharmaceutical manufacturers were putting two medications (most conspicuously, two antibiotics) in a fixed ratio into a single tablet or capsule and proclaiming great resultant advantages for the prescribing physician. These combinations appealed to the doctor who was too busy or too lazy to decide just what medications, and in what proportions, a particular patient needed. Most of these combinations have, quite properly, been removed from the prescription list. But the F.D.A.'s objection to the use of TMP-SMZ as a specific for chronic bacterial prostatitis—when it has already approved the combination for less well-defined conditions—has no rational basis.

In the United States a licensed physician can prescribe any approved drug for any ailment that he thinks it may alleviate or cure. But if he does so beyond the "indications" that the F.D.A. and a majority of his fellow specialists have approved, he does so at the risk of his colleagues' censure and perhaps a malpractice suit. Such risks seem negligible for a urologist who prescribes TMP-SMZ for recurrent bacterial prostatitis, since the F.D.A. approval states that it is "primarily for cystitis" (infections of the bladder) and kidney infections. That word "primarily" gives the doctor an out if he chooses to regard the prostate as covered under the previous wording, "for the treatment of chronic urinary tract infections . . . or infections associated with urinary tract complications such as obstruction." For an infected and inflamed prostate is certain to produce some obstruction of the urinary tract, and if the infection is chronic or recurrent, so much the worse.

Dr. Meares may have been the first but he is by no means the only eminent American urologist to put a liberal rather than a literal construction on the F.D.A. wording, and to use TMP-SMZ for many patients with chronic bacterial prostatitis. Neither he nor any other investigative physician can claim 100 percent cures, but the results are dramatically superior to those achieved with any other form of treatment for this baffling disorder.

In his first major investigation of the value of TMP-SMZ against laboratory-proved bacterial prostatitis, Dr. Meares treated thirteen volunteers aged twenty-four to sixty-four. They were given two tablets of the 80-400 mg. combination twice daily, one hour before meals, for fourteen days. Two patients may be said to have been cured, in that they were relieved of their symptoms during the treatment and had no recurrence as long as they could be followed. Nine were definitely improved, showing no symptoms and having a sterile prostate at the end of treatment, but they had relapses within five days to four months. One of the relapsing patients was infected with no fewer than four kinds of bacteria, one of which was knocked out completely by the treatment, while the other three reappeared. Two patients showed no improvement, which was surprising because both were infected with a strain of the common colon bacteria. Only one patient had to stop treatment because of an undesirable side effect, a measles-like rash that appeared when he had been on the drug for ten days. This was cured in a week with a common oral antihistamine.

These results were sufficiently encouraging for Dr. Meares and other urologists to undertake more extensive trials. Dr. George W. Drach, of the University of Arizona College of Medicine at Tucson, treated twenty-four patients with the same dosage of TMP-SMZ, but continued it for twenty-eight days. An unusual proportion of his patients were in the younger age ranges: one was under nineteen, and eleven others were under fifty; the remaining twelve were aged fifty to seventy-nine. Again there were more different kinds of infecting bacteria than there were patients: thirty-six varieties of microbes among the twenty-four men, and among them they had previously had a total of forty-five courses of antibiotic therapy. Data for six patients were inadequate, so Dr. Drach reported only on his results with eighteen. Of these he rated six (or 33 percent) as cured, since they had no relapses for as long as they could be followed, while twelve (the remaining 67 percent) suffered recurrences. Like other investigators, Dr. Drach found that certain of the less common microbes were the most resistant to treatment, and therefore most likely to produce relapses. (The blue-pus organism appeared to be completely resistant.)

At the Frederiksberg Hospital in Copenhagen, Dr. Mogens L. Nielsen and his colleagues worked with a quite different group of patients, consisting of nineteen men and six women. Sixteen of the men were over sixty, and all of them had benign prostatic

"Male Trouble"   Gilbert Cant

Septra ;   Bactrim   =   TMP - SMZ

Trimethoprim (TMP) 80 mg
Sulfamethoxazole (SMZ) 400 mg

Prostatitis = Inflammation [Acute & Chronic]
Prostatosis = Diseased (unknown cause)

Palpation — feeling for abnormal indication

E - coli = Colon bacilli (rectal), causes
80% of acute prostatitis

"Congestive Prosatitis" — from dramatic change
in sexual frequency : Unlikely theory

BPH = Benign Prostatic Hypertrophy

Adenoma = glandular tumor

TUR = Transurethral Resection (Resectoscope)
[c̄ electric cautery] ... for < 75g. growth
cyrosurgery c̄ Liq N$_2$

K.K.H.

Prostate regions : ①Periurethral glands surround urethra : ②transition
zone extends to : ③ Peripheral zone.
Per McLean in late 70's publications :
Prostate size constant from puberty to ca. 50 yrs, then
enlarges in 2/3's of men = BPH
Growth in 40's often in Periurethral glands.
Growth in 50's usually transition zone.

From

Barry B. Holmes

hypertrophy, some with other complications. The three younger men (aged twenty-eight to thirty-eight) had a narrowing of the urethra from other causes; in all nineteen male patients the urinary channel was constricted. The six women were not treated for prostatitis, which is extremely rare in women, but for urinary tract infections originating in the kidneys, complicated in most cases by the presence of kidney stones. The Danes had thought that with urethral constriction from any cause, relapses were almost inevitable, especially among the older patients. They were gratified to see that in nineteen cases (fourteen men and five women), they were able to suppress the infection for as long as three months with the small maintenance dose of a single 80-400 mg. tablet twice daily.

More and more urologists are coming to believe that with this modest dose of TMP-SMZ, or even a single tablet daily, which is well tolerated by the great majority of patients, it should be possible to control chronic bacterial prostatitis as effectively as most cases of diabetes are controlled by medication, and hypothyroidism by a thyroid hormone preparation. It is estimated that despite the slowdown imposed by the F.D.A., no fewer than two-thirds of all victims of chronic bacterial prostatitis in the United States have already had some treatment with TMP-SMZ, but it seems certain that only a minute fraction of these patients were treated long enough or intensively enough.

Dr. Scott of Johns Hopkins sums it up: "I believe we really can cure not only acute but chronic prostatitis. The trouble is that too many patients are not treated long enough. First there must be an accurate diagnosis based on identifying the cultured bacteria, then intensive treatment directed specifically at this organism. Finally, continuance with suppressive therapy, with whatever is the safest and most active drug available."

It is not yet certain that TMP-SMZ is as nearly ideal a treatment for chronic prostatitis as some of its advocates believe, but there was a disturbing time lag between the exploration and reporting of its usefulness in Europe and its approval for any purpose in the United States, and specific approval for its use in prostatis is still to come. As *The New York Times* noted on March 2, 1976, in a survey of American medicine, "What seems needed . . . is a better mechanism for monitoring medical progress outside this country and for taking advantage of foreign experience to help validate medicines and medical procedures that may be useful here."

Chapter

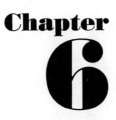

Prostatosis or What?

The unknown or unidentified disorder is often more frightening than the known and identified, even though it may be medically less serious. The victims of acute and chronic bacterial prostatitis can usually get an accurate diagnosis of their condition and in most cases they can count on being cured or obtaining substantial relief. There remains a third class of prostatic disorders in which the unknown is still an extremely important element. Many urologists, especially the younger investigators and practitioners, call this condition "prostatosis." Whereas the Greek suffix -*itis* indicates inflammation, the suffix -*osis* means simply a state or condition, and in medicine this is applied only to a diseased or unhealthy state or condition. (If all were normal, there would be no point in mentioning it.) One of the puzzling unknowns about this condition is why it seems to attack almost as many people as the identifiable forms of bacterial prostatitis.

The victims of prostatosis suffer from some but not all of the same symptoms as those associated with bacterial prostatitis. The majority complain of pain

in the lower back and perineal region; they are likely
to have a burning sensation in the urethra during
urination or after ejaculation, and to suffer from urinary urgency or frequency or both. They seldom report chills or fever, and virtually none of them have
a history of previous, confirmed infections of the urinary tract. They show no evidence of true prostatic
enlargement, although some may complain of tenderness or pain when the physician's finger palpates
the gland. The most conspicuous difference between
the signs of infectious prostatitis and of prostatosis is
that laboratory cultures yield no harvests of infecting
bacteria. If any microbes are grown from the urine
specimens they are likely to be few in number and
belong to species that are regarded as normally harm-
less inhabitants of the genitourinary system. Attempts to identify and convict viruses as the cause of
prostatosis have failed.

Because no infectious agent can be identified in so
many cases of prostatic inflammation, some medical
scientists call the condition "abacterial prostatitis,"
and one has coined the term "nonprostatitis prostatitis," which recalls George Orwell's Newspeak. Although some patients report feeling improved after
treatment with an antibiotic, usually tetracycline,
there is no certainty that this is because of an antibacterial effect. The benefit, if any, is likely to be of
short duration, and some specialists believe that it is
more psychological than physiological.

Many cases of prostatosis are in a category that
urologists of another, older school call "congestive
prostatitis." Dr. Philip R. Roen, a respected and suc-

cessful Manhattan urologist, believes a common cause to be "poor sexual practices." The glandular cells, he points out, secrete prostatic fluid more or less continuously. This is expelled by muscular contraction into the urethra at the time of orgasmic ejaculation. He contends that if the prostatic fluid is denied such a natural outlet, it accumulates, deteriorates, and causes congestion, perhaps with inflammation, in the secreting glands. (The adolescent's wet dreams might be regarded as one of nature's defenses against such a condition, although other explanations are equally plausible.) Dr. Roen calls congestive prostatitis "priests' disease," because he has observed it in a number of seminarians and members of celibate orders.

Paradoxically, congestive prostatitis may, according to Dr. Roen, result from the opposite cause: too frequent excitation and ejaculation (whether by masturbation or any form of intercourse), thus putting an excessive burden on the secretory parts of the prostate—in effect, demanding that they work overtime. It may also occur, says Dr. Roen, when a man changes his pattern of sexual activity abruptly, either from abstinence to satiety or vice versa. And although the disorder may appear in a teen-aged youth, it becomes more common with advancing years.

Whatever the cause or causes of congestive prostatitis, it seems unlikely that it can be explained by anything as undefinable as "poor sexual practices." And although Dr. Roen understandably advocates moderation, this is almost equally undefinable. For at least ten thousand years men have had infinitely various rates of sexual frequency, ranging from the zero of total abstinence (voluntary or involuntary) to orgiastic satiation. The prostate, despite its many elements of mystery, is one of the innumerable organs into which nature has built an incredibly wide tolerance for variations in excitation, secretion, and excretion. There is not enough evidence in the medical archives to relate activity on any band of the human sex spectrum directly to congestive prostatitis, or to any form of prostatosis.

What is certain is that the victim of this disorder (or group of disorders) suffers many of the miseries of his peers who have diagnosable disease, but has less hope of obtaining lasting relief. Dr. Roen believes that many men are helped by a change in sexual practice; it is likely that the doctor's own reassuring personality may be the most effective item in this prescription.

For the patient whose congestion is attributable to near or total abstinence, massage of the gland by the doctor's gloved finger often produces relief. This is professionally ascribed to emptying of the stagnating prostatic fluid which is then expelled through the urethra, relieving intraglandular pressure. This obviously is a form of sexual stimulation which may in itself be satisfying, so a man, especially an older, long-married man, who experiences marital difficulties at the same time as his prostatosis develops, may find double relief in prostatic massage. In most cases there is no medical reason not to suggest trying masturbation, though the doctor who will recommend this to his patient of his own accord is rare indeed.

One common prescription for prostatosis, however defined, is the sitz bath. The warmth itself is comforting, and seems to relieve much of the aching in the lower back and perineal region, although no direct effect on the prostate's secretory mechanism is apparent.

None of these palliative measures will satisfy most victims of prostatosis. And—most emphatically—these patients are not suitable candidates for surgery. They are among the most persistent of all doctor shoppers, forever hoping that the next urologist will have a more definitive and effective prescription. At the end of this peripatetic process, many fall victim to another abuse and the worst of prescriptions: quackery. Urologists who are as frustrated and almost as disappointed as their patients by treatment failures can only hope that some effective medication will soon be synthesized in the laboratories of today's alchemists.

Chapter

BPH: Benign Enlargement

In medical language "benign" means nonmalignant and that almost invariably means simply noncancerous. Benign overgrowth or enlargement of the prostate, which doctors call benign prostatic hypertrophy or hyperplasia, and refer to as BPH, is certainly not cancerous. Yet although it is benign it is not necessarily a trivial complaint. BPH can set off a chain reaction of other genitourinary problems. When the condition is accurately diagnosed and its severity established, it is often a signal for the surgeon to intervene, as the development of palliative treatments with medication has been hampered by the scarcity of promising pharmaceuticals.

Any abnormal swelling or internal enlargement is called a tumor. To distinguish between different types, tumors are described by adding the Greek suffix -*oma* to the name of the overgrowing tissue. Since the prostate is a gland, or *aden* in Greek, overgrowth or enlargement of the prostate is an adenoma. The patient who hears this word exchanged between his doctor and an assistant should not be alarmed. BPH is an adenoma but not a malignant or cancerous tumor.

Although these important facts are clear, much else about BPH is either unclear or unknown. For example, why should infectious prostatitis become less common among men of advancing age, while BPH occurs with increasing frequency? No one knows. Some authorities consider it a natural part of the aging process, since it eventually affects 50 percent of men who live much beyond the age of fifty. Dr. Roen disputes this, contending that BPH cannot be normal or natural, because 50 percent of men do not develop it.

Some men who develop BPH remain totally unaware of any symptoms or discomfort. Dr. David A. Culp, head of the department of urology at the University of Iowa Hospitals and Clinics, says, "The enlarged prostate in and of itself produces few if any symptoms." But the prostate is not an independent organ and when it becomes enlarged it affects the urethra, which it enfolds, or the adjacent bladder neck.

Benign tumors may develop in almost any part of the body at any time of life, often with no explainable cause, but the prostate is unusual in its tendency for half or more of the gland to become enlarged without having suffered any apparent injury, either physical or chemical. One theory is that as man has prolonged his life span beyond what nature originally intended for him, many of the cells in the forward lobes of the prostate undergo a form of atrophy or wasting process, but instead of shrinking they expand and thus exert pressure upon adjacent areas. This "explanation" requires another to explain the atrophy, and one suggestion is that as a man grows older his prostate receives less and less testosterone from his testicles. But this is not true. So long as men remain healthy the great majority—as many as 80 percent, according to Dr. Martin A. Robbins, chief of urology at Sinai Hospital, Baltimore—continue to produce the same amount of testosterone well beyond middle life. They may do so until the age of seventy or perhaps beyond. Some investigators believe that since BPH cannot be directly related to a decrease in testosterone supply, it may be due to a change in the body's method of metabolizing this hormone. (Most of it is rapidly changed biochemically into a related and highly potent form, dihydrotestosterone.) Although researchers' theories differ in regard to the precise mechanisms involved, there is a fairly general consensus that BPH results from some hormonal imbalance.

The symptoms may develop so gradually that men who do not have regular and thorough physical examinations may neglect BPH for months or years. This is most likely to be true of the man whose only urinary disturbance is the need to void in the middle of the night; he is apt to dismiss this as part of the price of living to a ripe age. Such neglect is understandable if enlargement of the prostate causes only moderate obstruction of the urinary outlet at the bladder neck or just below it, for the bladder has a considerable capacity for adapting to the situation. It will perform an Atlas-style muscle-building feat to

strengthen its wall, and it will work harder to expel
urine against the increased resistance at or below its
outlet. As long as the muscles succeed in emptying
the bladder completely on each voiding, there will be
no retained urine to cause infection higher up the
urinary tract. The first evidence of this mild condition is found during a routine physical or perhaps an
examination for other, unrelated problems, when an
enlargement of the part of the prostate adjoining the
rectum is noticed. This condition is called "silent
prostatism."

If there is hypertrophy anywhere in the prostate,
the chances are that it will eventually progress to a
stage where it produces some of the symptoms of disease. These will be a reduction in the volume and
force of the urinary stream; difficulty in beginning to
urinate (sometimes inability to do so); and a feeling
that the bladder has not been emptied completely,
resulting in the need to urinate at short intervals. If
the urine retained in the bladder develops infection,
then the act of micturition (a synonym for urination,
favored by some urologists) becomes a painful process. If the discharge is slow as well as painful the condition is called strangury. And if the bladder neck or
the urethra is completely closed by enlargement of the
prostate, the effect is to produce strangulation of the
urinary tract.

Complete strangulation is a true medical emergency. The victim is most probably a man aged
seventy or older, who has neglected some urinary
difficulties for years because the severity of the symptoms increases gradually and insidiously, giving no

clear alarm signal. Naturally he has been unaware of the fact that during this period the muscles of his bladder wall have become exhausted from the constant stretching demanded of them. The muscle may have suffered partial ruptures producing pouches external to the bladder itself—diverticula, such as are found more often on the large bowel.

The man wakes in the middle of the night in acute agony. It is usually his wife who telephones the doctor and says, "You must come over at once. He can't bear it." The doctor is justified, this time, in declining to make a house call. Instead he orders the patient taken to the nearest hospital emergency room, and treats him there.

In such a case, with no evidence of an acute inflammatory infection, the urologist will not hesitate to catheterize his patient. And with his unbearable pain, the patient is not likely to demand reassurance about the procedure. He may be told just to take four deep breaths, and relax. The lubricated plastic tube is inserted through the urethra and threaded up into the bladder. This may be intensely uncomfortable for a minute or so but is far less distressing than the bladder pain it will relieve. The gush of dammed-up urine is immediate and gives immediate relief. If necessary, the catheter may be left in place for a day or two, for continued ease of voiding. Or if it is decided that the patient needs surgery, the catheter may remain in place for ten days to two weeks until he is in strong enough condition for a corrective operation.

Among younger men the symptoms of BPH are

often less severe and do not produce a crisis demanding instantaneous and direct relief. They do, however, require careful diagnosis. Dr. Culp says, "A large, benign prostate, simply because of its size, may produce perineal aching or pain." Such pain may suggest totally different diseases and thus lead to misdiagnosis. Reverse flow, or impedance of outward flow, from the kidneys through the ureters to the bladder can produce a watery swelling of the kidneys similar to that caused by gastrointestinal disease. This is marked by nausea, vomiting, loss of appetite and weight, and a general feeling of lethargy and malaise. If the condition is further complicated by infection, it will produce chills and fever and pain in various parts of the body.

The most important distinction to be made, says Dr. Culp, is between acute inflammatory (infectious) disease and purely physical obstruction: "Disastrous results may follow surgery in patients whose disease is inflammatory rather than obstructive"—for the reason already noted, that surgical intervention may spread an active infection.

Dr. Culp divides the diagnostic procedures for BPH into four categories: 1) physical, 2) laboratory, 3) radiographic, and 4) instrumental.

The most obvious physical findings relate to the size, shape, consistency, and tenderness of the gland upon rectal palpation. During this examination the doctor presses against the gland repeatedly, firmly but gently, to propel prostatic fluid into the urethra. Microscopic examination of cultures from the squeezed-out fluid will show whether or not infectious organisms are present: BPH by itself does not add bacteria or abnormal components resulting from infection (such as an excess of white blood cells) to the prostatic fluid. Further laboratory tests are useful mainly to show whether BPH has caused sufficient backing up of urine into the bladder to promote an ascending infection, which must be treated with medication (probably the sulfas) as already described.

Radiologic (X-ray) tests for determining how far BPH has developed and the extent of its obstructive effects on the urinary system are numerous and technically complex. Most involve the injection of a radiopaque solution containing an element such as iodine, which blocks the passage of X rays almost as though the vessels containing it were solid bone. Therefore they show up in contrasting white or pale tones on the X-ray negative. The procedure, called an intravenous urogram, is essentially the same as the intravenous pyelogram for suspected kidney disease. The dye is injected into an arm vein and travels through the blood stream. A series of films will show the kidneys and ureters and whether they have been damaged by a reverse flow of urine. Next the bladder is outlined, to reveal the degree of its enlargement and the possible presence of diverticula. At its neck, the obstructing overgrown prostate appears, not as sharply defined as the other organs, but in most cases clearly enough to give the urologist a valuable indication of the location and approximate size of the hypertrophy.

By both laboratory and X-ray tests, the urologist will be careful to rule out any form of kidney disease that might produce confusing symptoms, notably anemia. And the X rays will show whether there are stones (calculi) in the kidneys, the bladder, or the prostate itself.

The most conclusive evidence of BPH comes when the patient is in the "lithotomy" (stone-cutting) position, similar to that for childbirth, for internal examination with the cystoscope. This is not a simple tube, like the catheter, but a more sophisticated device, with which the physician literally looks inside the bladder. Some urologists commonly put their patients under general anesthesia for this procedure; others prefer a spinal anesthetic; and still others try to avoid the use of any anesthetic. The choice depends not only upon the physician's preference but upon the physical and emotional state of the patient. Most men have from boyhood a horror of having any instrument inserted in the urethra, since they are aware of its tenderness near its outlet, the only part with which they are familiar. But the urethra is remarkably distensible, and will accept the insertion of a suitably lubricated instrument up to at least the thickness of a lead pencil, or as much as one centimeter (3/8 inch) in diameter. If the patient is psychologically prepared for the procedure and is convinced that if he relaxes he will feel nothing worse than moderate discomfort, he can undergo both catheterization and cystoscopy without marked distress. The patient who finds it unbearably painful is the one who has not been psychologically prepared, and who becomes tense at the thought, let alone the sight, of the instrument.

Catheterization is performed after the patient, either before anesthesia or without it, has been encouraged to urinate energetically and thus empty his bladder as completely as possible. The catheter is then threaded gently through the urethra, past the constriction at about the level of the prostate, and into the bladder. In many cases the incompleteness of earlier voiding becomes evident in a brisk flow of urine that emerges as soon as the catheter enters the bladder.

The catheter is withdrawn and replaced by the cystoscope—one of the triumphs of modern fiber-optics. Although instruments and techniques vary in detail, in most cases a thin tube, capable of transmitting light around bends and with a bulb the size of a rice grain at its end, is inserted through the urethra. With this the urologist can directly inspect the interior of the bladder. This examination will show whether its muscles, having first grown and strengthened themselves to propel urine against increased resistance at the bladder neck or in the urethra, have by now become fatigued and flaccid. Depending upon the severity and duration of the strain imposed on the bladder, its walls may show small cracks between their muscular fibers, then little pouches or "saccules," and, finally, larger pockets or diverticula. At any of these stages the bladder wall may be streaked with irregular lines, like wrinkled skin.

One form of the endoscope ("look inside") instrument has what are in effect two telescopes in a single tube, aimed at different angles for better visualization of the bladder neck and urethra as distinct from the interior of the bladder itself. Whatever type of endoscope is used it should show the urologist whether hypertrophy of the prostate's median lobe has obstructed the bladder neck. This will tend to obscure his view and may have created a ball-valve mechanism that was responsible for the urinary retention.

As it is withdrawn slightly the endoscope will disclose the condition of the lateral lobes. These are prime suspects for overgrowth, as they encroach upon the urethra in the zone of the verumontanum. If these lobes have enlarged more or less symmetrically they will have squeezed the urethra into a narrow channel, like a hose that becomes flat when empty. This condition also results in a lengthening of the urethra, as the prostate tends to enlarge simultaneously in the vertical as well as the horizontal dimension. Whichever lobes are enlarged, these will be the target for the surgeon seeking to effect a definitive cure of BPH.

Regardless of its detailed effects upon the urinary system, BPH may cause intense aches and pains merely from the increased bulk of the prostate. The volume of the overgrowth varies enormously with both the duration of the process and unpredictable differences between patients. With reasonably prompt medical attention, the disorder should be detected and treated before the gland has more than doubled its original size. In these cases the patient may obtain surgical cure of his hypertrophy by the most modern and least radical of prostate operations, the transurethral resection, or TUR (see Chapter Eight). This should not impair his sexual function or even his fertility.

In neglected or extreme cases the enlargement may be much more dramatic. Grossly hypertrophied prostates have been reported to be as big as a grapefruit or a coconut. These and similar, less hyperbolic comparisons are unscientific and imprecise, but they are clear in one respect: they indicate beyond question that the patient should undergo surgery by one of the more radical procedures.

It would obviously be desirable to treat the enlarged prostate with medication rather than surgery, and physicians have been trying to do so for almost half a century. Dr. Andrew Sporer, of Martland Hospital in Newark, New Jersey, says that while the methods were based on seemingly valid theories, all yielded only unsatisfactory results until Soviet investigators tested an antibiotic generally used against fungal infections. In the United States it is called candicidin (in the USSR, levorin). Dr. Sporer's group found that candicidin produced "over-all improvement" in 78 percent of patients who took two capsules three times daily for three to seven months. All the most familiar symptoms—nocturia, urgency, frequency, intermittency, hesitancy, and dribbling— were relieved to a significant degree. In cases where surgery was later considered necessary it was found that the enlarged gland had shrunk substantially during medical treatment. Urologists at other medical centers have reported similarly encouraging results and the manufacturers of candicidin have asked the Food and Drug Administration to approve its use in BPH. But candicidin remains in a bureaucratic limbo comparable to that of TMP-SMZ.

Chapter

Surgery

If we set aside clearly identifiable cases of acute or chronic infectious prostatitis and the vaguely defined conditions grouped as prostatosis, there are two principal disorders of the gland for which surgery is likely to be recommended and may be mandatory. These are BPH and cancer. Surgery is occasionally performed for chronic prostatitis, but never during a period of active infection. And even then there is some dispute among prostatologists as to its advisability and effectiveness.

There are four major types of operation, and since they may be recommended in cases of either benign enlargement or cancer, they are described here in the order of how "radical" they are generally considered. (There is some disagreement among surgeons about the order in which they should be rated.) The extent of the operation is not necessarily an indicator of the severity of the underlying disease. It may reflect simply the size and the direction of spread of a benign overgrowth, or the surgeon's preferred method of treating a particular condition.

The earliest surgical procedure for prostatic disease was the most drastic of all: a perineal incision for insertion of a crude instrument to remove the entire gland. This may have been performed two thousand or more years ago, when it must have been a truly agonizing procedure, with no general anesthesia and only the analgesic (pain-reducing) benefit from a knockout dose of some alcoholic beverage to ease the patient's pangs. Today, anesthesia and enormously refined techniques have revolutionized the experience of the patient undergoing prostatic surgery.

The most modern and sophisticated form of operation for prostatic disorders is the transurethral resection ("cutting out through the urethra"), or TUR. It is technically a major operation, with the patient usually under general anesthesia, although some medical centers prefer to use deep spinal anesthesia. (The choice will depend largely upon the patient's age and general physical condition, and upon the surgeon's estimate of how long the operation will take. If this is an hour or longer, the spinal is usually preferred.) Either way, the TUR is the least traumatic procedure for the patient, since it does not require an external incision. Recovery is usually smooth and complete within two weeks, the patient's principal complaint being that the catheter to drain urine past the surgical wound in the urethra must remain in place to permit healing without infection; and the TUR has the advantage over alternative operations that it does not usually reduce sexual potency. Indeed, it may increase potency or restore lost sexual ability (see Chapter Ten).

In selecting patients with BPH as suitable candidates for a TUR operation the urologic surgeon is guided largely by the size of the overgrowth. The consensus is that for this procedure to be practicable and effective, the prostate must not have overgrown to a weight greater than 75 grams (about 2½ ounces), or about the size of an average breakfast egg.

Although simple for the patient, the TUR is one of the most exactingly difficult procedures for the urologic surgeon to learn and to perform successfully. Developing this skill and expertise may require serving for years as the chief assistant to a senior surgeon and participating in as many as a hundred operations.

The TUR begins in much the same way as the cystoscopy described earlier. With the anesthetized patient in the lithotomy position, the surgeon threads a catheter up the urethra. Since the patient has emptied his bladder as completely as possible before the anesthesia, there is usually no great gush of retained urine at this stage. However, there is almost certain to be at least a moderate flow, the evidence of some retention. Next, a resectoscope is inserted in the urethra. This is a "look-see, cutting-out" instrument. There are some variations between different models, and differences in the details of design, but the basic principle is always the same. The light transmitted along the fiberoptic path enables the urologist to see the tissues around the tip of the resectoscope. There he also has a minuscule knife or cutting wire, or (more likely nowadays) an electric cautery.

What the surgeon does with his resectoscope depends largely, of course, upon what X rays and other diagnostic tests have revealed. But even with a clear case of BPH, he must still identify visually which parts of which lobes have become enlarged and are encroaching on other organs or vessels. He then cuts these with his knife or wire, or cauterizes them electrically. Many particles are removed during the operation. Some that are difficult to remove at this time may be left, with the knowledge that within a day or so they will be flushed out by the prostatic or urinary flows, or will be destroyed by the body's normal clearance processes.

For overgrowths of moderate size, some innovative urologists interested in the ultramodern technique of cryosurgery (freezing the tissues by an injection of liquid nitrogen at a temperature of $-196°C$.) have attempted to relieve BPH with this noncutting technique. Unfortunately, some of the earlier investigators proceeded most enthusiastically and perhaps prematurely, so that the results were unsatisfactory and the procedure fell into some disrepute. But with recent improvements in both instrumentation and surgical skill, it is now possible to use this procedure in selected cases. In cryosurgery for BPH the surgeon freezes a little ball of the hyperplastic tissue, thus killing it, or, as the doctors say, inducing necrosis. When this dead tissue is allowed to thaw out, after only a few minutes, some may promptly emerge in liquefied form through the instrument already in place, while some will remain in the prostate. Whatever remains will be sloughed off by the body through its natural cleansing operations, and will be eliminated through the urine over a period of probably two or three days. As is often the case with innovative techniques, the use of cryosurgery for relief of BPH has been for some years a matter of dispute among the experts, and is likely to remain so for some years more. Although generally considered still in the experimental stage, it appears to be a moderately promising alternative for carefully selected patients treated only by the most carefully trained cryosurgeons.

Although the TUR is a triumph of surgical ingenuity, its results in cases of chronic prostatitis are not so predictably rewarding as in operations for BPH. The outcome does not always justify the patient's optimism or the surgeon's expenditure of time, skill, and patience. At Stanford University Hospital only about one third of the patients operated upon in this manner were cured, in the sense that they had sterile urine and prostatic secretion cultures for many months or years. It is true that of the two thirds who were not cured, none was considered to have been made worse—a tribute to the skill of the operating surgeon. But this majority of patients resumed their previous pattern of persistent reinfection, though possibly after longer periods of remission, with the type of microbe that had caused their original chronic prostatitis. Urologic surgeons in other medical centers have reported considerably higher cure rates, but these investigators were not always able to show that there had indeed been an earlier bacterial prostatitis. The patients may have been suffering from the condition described as prostatosis.

The third condition for which a TUR is sometimes advised is cancer of the prostate. When this procedure is considered for malignant disease, the surgeon must be convinced that he is dealing with its earliest form, a discrete group of cancer cells not more than one centimeter (3/8 inch) in diameter. The choice of a TUR for even so small and early a cancer is still debatable.

If a patient's BPH is so extensive, or takes such a conformation, that it cannot be adequately treated by a TUR, the alternative is a "radical" prostatectomy. We do not need to engage here in the endless "how radical is 'radical'?" controversy, which began before 1900 and bears a remarkable resemblance to the disputes among breast surgeons as to how radical a mastectomy for cancer of the female breast should be. The two major surgical treatments for severe BPH are called suprapubic and retropubic prostatectomies. Despite the literal meaning of the word prostatectomy—cutting out the prostate—these operations usually are not quite so drastic. For both types of operation similar incisions are made: on the lower pelvis, over or near the "symphysis pubis," or pubic bone. The essential difference between the two procedures is in the direction taken by the scalpel beyond the incision. In the suprapubic form the surgeon goes straight ahead and cuts into the bladder neck to gain access to hypertrophic tissue there and thence to the prostate below. In the retropubic form the scalpel is directed at a lower angle, to avoid the bladder neck and its nerve and muscle attachments, and so enable the surgeon to operate on the prostate alone.

A third open surgical approach to the prostate, whether for BPH or a more serious condition, is through a perineal incision between the anus and the scrotum. This has been, until recently, the preferred route for a truly total prostatectomy in which the entire gland, with its capsule, is removed. Some surgeons now choose the retropubic route instead. Since they remove the whole prostate along with the seminal vesicles, this kind of radical surgery is equivalent to a total prostatectomy, however defined.

Many medical considerations must be taken into account in determining which of these surgical approaches will be used. Since most patients are men of relatively advanced years, they may have disorders or diseases totally unrelated to the prostate but important in relation to any kind of surgery—such as diabetes or a cardiovascular condition. Many of them will also have regrettably obese abdomens, which make the suprapubic or retropubic operation more difficult. Patients of any age who have emphysema or obstructive pulmonary disease are also poor candidates for the abdominal approach. The size of a prostatic overgrowth is an important element in determining whether or not a TUR is feasible or desirable, but if the hypertrophy is too large to permit a TUR, then size alone will not have great influence on the choice between the different open surgical approaches.

If the X rays and other diagnostic procedures in-

dicate that the hypertrophy results from the enlargement of either the lateral or the median lobes and
their projection upward into the bladder neck, then
the surgeon will almost certainly use the suprapubic
route, since this enables him to reach the urinary system at precisely this point. This approach has the
further advantage that, by exposing the bladder to
the scalpel, the surgeon is able to correct any associated disease areas in the bladder itself.

If the preoperative evidence indicates that the
lateral lobes have grown principally around the
urethra and do not project upward, the surgeon is
more likely to choose the retropubic approach, by
which he is able to reach the prostatic urethra itself
without necessarily entering the bladder. This has
the advantage of making the prostatic urethra and its
immediately adjacent tissues more directly visible,
and therefore more readily operable. Its disadvantage
is the risk of damage to a complex system of blood
vessels.

Both the suprapubic and retropubic approaches
have the advantage over the perineal of not necessarily causing impotence. Whether or not the patient
retains potency after his operation depends to some
extent upon the skill of the surgeon in avoiding damage to nerve and muscle structures involved in the
contractions necessary at the time of erection and
later of orgasm, and partly upon the extent to which
these structures were already impaired.

According to many authorities, patients complain
of impotence following about 25 percent of suprapubic and retropubic operations, but this does not

mean that the operations are the cause of the impotence. In most cases the true cause is unknown. In many it is clearly psychogenic, reflecting an irrational but understandable feeling of having somehow been emasculated. Or the complaint is used as an excuse for avoiding intercourse with a partner who no longer seems desirable. The one change that is certain to follow either operation is that the recovered patient will no longer have a discernible ejaculate at orgasm. This has nothing to do with the ability to reach orgasm, but only with fertility (see Chapter Ten).

The perineal route has advantages for the surgeon in greater accessibility of the prostate as approached from below, but the great disadvantage from the viewpoint of many patients in the younger age ranges (under sixty-five or seventy) that it carries a relatively high risk of inducing impotence and to some degree of incontinence after recovery.

These procedures sound formidable and perhaps frightening, but for most patients it is preferable to undergo any one of them, in skilled surgical hands, rather than continue suffering from increasingly severe BPH. In the early days of prostatectomy the operation caused or hastened the death of 25 percent of patients. This mortality has been reduced today, in the better medical centers, to less than one percent. The man who is fortunate enough to have no coincidental impairment of his health and has an operation for BPH is likely to emerge greatly improved in both mind and body, genuinely glad he followed his doctor's advice.

A friend of mine, an author who normally likes to see his name in print as often as possible but prefers to remain anonymous in this context, was sixty-two when he found himself suffering from the symptoms of BPH, which in his case included the near-impossibility of sexual intercourse. Before surgery, he was able to enjoy sexual intercourse only about once a month, and each time dreaded the burning urethral pain that followed orgasm. He had a retropubic prostatectomy, during which the surgeon removed tissue which he described as "about the size of an orange." My friend made a complete recovery within less than a month, and shortly thereafter looked younger than he had in years. He reported that he was not only free of pain and discomfort, but was thoroughly enjoying intercourse two or three times a week.

Any surgery on the prostate, from a TUR to the more drastic radical and total prostatectomies, is likely to be what doctors call an elective procedure, meaning that its timing is not an emergency matter but can safely be postponed for three to four weeks. This leads to an important and fortunate cautionary note. The patient undergoing such surgery is likely to lose considerable blood—less in a TUR than in the other operations—and may need a transfusion. Serious reactions from mismatched blood, or from donor blood infected with hepatitis virus, are among the commonest causes of death following surgery. Therefore a patient who is well enough to give blood should be his own donor and provide two or perhaps three pints two to four weeks before the operation.

No one was ever poisoned by a transfusion of his own blood.

Physicians who do not practice surgery, and even many surgeons who are highly skilled and successful with the scalpel, would strongly prefer to see BPH, chronic prostatitis, and the earliest stages of cancer treated medicinally rather than surgically. This is not yet in sight, although more effective medical treatments seem certain to be perfected in the future.

Chapter
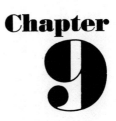

Cancer and Its Treatment

Every man who has ever had any disorder of the prostate, however benign, is likely to envisage cancer as the dark at the end of the urethral tunnel. Since the prostate consists primarily of glandular tissue, cancer in this organ is technically known as an adenocarcinoma. Like other carcinomas, it can exhibit remarkable differences in the ways in which it develops and—most important—in the speed at which it may progress.

So much publicity has been given—with the best of intentions—to the problems and dangers of malignancies that many people now have what can only be called cancerophobia. Some of this has developed out of the campaigns to have women examine their own breasts for lumps, in the hope that this procedure will lead to early detection of mammary cancer and minimize the surgery it may require. In the case of the male prostate, whose glandular tissue closely resembles the breast tissue of the female, no such popular concern has yet been generated, although enough cancerophobia to lead to regular checkups among the male population would certainly be beneficial.

The prostate is placed so that a man cannot perform an effective self-examination, and even if he could, he would not have sufficient skill to interpret the feel of the posterior surface of the prostate. But for most men there are plenty of opportunities for physical examinations, which will include the simple rectal palpation by the physician's gloved finger. The examination is desirable for men of any age, but it is imperative for those aged fifty or over. One proof of this is a set of figures supplied by Dr. Gerald P. Murphy for Western New York State: among hundreds of cases of prostate cancer diagnosed in that region in recent years, fewer than one percent have been detected in the early stages, when they would be operable and most likely curable.

The National Cancer Institute's projection for 1976 was that there would be about 60,000 new cases of prostatic cancer diagnosed in the United States. The Institute also predicted 19,300 deaths resulting from this disease. This latter figure may be an underestimate, since even now many physicians, especially those in general practice in small communities, are reluctant to record cancer as a cause of death. Just as no one yet knows why an otherwise healthy and normal prostate tends to hypertrophy with advancing years, so no one knows why the prostate is so commonly the site of malignant disease. Several types of cancer are now attributable to disease-causing (mostly chemical and radioactive) substances in the environment, but cancer of the prostate is not among these. The incidence, or at least the reported incidence, has increased so markedly in recent years that prostatic cancer is now displacing cancer of the colon, and ranks second only to lung cancer associated with cigarette smoking as the leading cause of cancer deaths among males.

There are three ways in which prostatic cancer can be detected in its earliest stages. The first is from the rectal examination, when the physician finds a nodule or nodules on the part of the prostate that projects into the rectum. He cannot at first be certain whether these represent cancerous nodules or merely stones (calculi). At this point the second detection medium, the needle biopsy, comes into play: the removal with a heavy needle of a tiny piece of tissue, so that the pathologist with his microscope can determine whether or not cancerous cells are present. The third means of early detection is simply fortuitous: it results from a patient's having had a TUR for BPH. As a precaution, a sample of the tissue removed in this operation is routinely subjected to microscopic examination, and it may show the presence of cancer cells, even though the disease is still in such an early stage as to be otherwise undetectable. With the passage of time, cancer in the prostate may extend through most of the gland, and eventually through its tough retaining capsule to adjacent tissues in the urethra and bladder or rectum. Later it may metastasize—that is, colonize, or spread to more distant parts of the body.

Since the type of treatment indicated for prostatic cancer varies widely with the stage at which the disease is discovered, it became apparent about 1950 that a system of classifying these steps was necessary.

In 1956 Dr. Willet F. Whitmore, Jr., of the Memorial Sloan-Kettering Cancer Center, proposed such a system, dividing prostatic cancer into four categories: A, B, C, and D.

Stage A cancer of the prostate is confined within the gland itself. In Stage B, according to some authorities, the cancer has spread but still only inside the capsule, while others consider that it may have protruded through part of the prostate capsule but not yet invaded other organs. In Stage C it has reached farther out, but still only to adjacent organs, notably the seminal vesicles. And in Stage D the cancer cells have migrated, perhaps through the lymphatic system, and established colonies (metastases) in the pelvis and eventually beyond that to the lungs and bones.

At first glance it would seem that discovery of Stage A disease, confined within the prostate and causing no detectable symptoms, should make it easy for doctor and patient to agree that surgery is desirable, and dictate the extent of the operation to be performed. But it is not as simple as that. Even after a repeat biopsy, detailed laboratory work, and perhaps X-ray or other tests, specialists cannot predict what course the disease will take. For no less important than the *stage* of a prostatic cancer is its *grade*— a term used to indicate whether it is so mildly active that it will grow slowly if at all, or a hyperactive variety that may reach Stage B within a month.

Some men who have refused surgery when Stage A was diagnosed, or who have not been operated on for other reasons, have lived as long as fifteen years with no obvious symptoms of disease. Since the majority have been sixty-two or older at the time of diagnosis, most of them have lived out a normal life span and died of some unrelated cause, usually heart disease. This has prompted a few—but very few—urologists to suggest leaving Stage A cancer alone for a while, taking a wait-and-see attitude. Dr. Hugh J. Jewett, emeritus professor of urology at Johns Hopkins, points out that this is like playing Russian roulette.

Dr. Jewett suggests that Stage A cancers be subdivided into two grades, 1 and 2, the former being the less likely to progress to more serious disease. But at the current stage of research, the most expert cytologist (cell specialist) cannot predict from the appearance of these cells, in the first specimen submitted to him, how they will behave in the next few months or even weeks. To see the pattern and establish the grade, follow-up tests of tissues and cells are necessary, and the time lost between tests is the Russian roulette period.

So the most experienced prostatologists disagree. There is no consensus as to what if anything should be done about a single, small focus of Stage A—presumably Grade 1—tumor. The compromise in which a fair number concur is that this requires a TUR, performed in the hope that all the cancer tissue, being so neatly confined, can be removed.

But despite Dr. Jewett's colorful analogy, there are eminent specialists who believe that Stage A-1 can be merely observed, at least for a while, thus sparing the patient any surgery. The Memorial Sloan-Kettering Cancer Center in New York has a

reputation for using the most radical forms of treatment—largely because so many patients are not re-
ferred there until their disease is far advanced, and
usually not until other physicians have tried vainly
to treat the condition. But at Memorial, Dr. Whitmore says that a patient with Stage A (presumably
Grade 1) cancer can be spared immediate treatment,
and perhaps spared indefinitely, if he will cooperate
with his physician and have a reexamination every
two or three months. His disease may prove to be of
the type that remains latent for many years. Dr.
Whitmore points out that a relatively young man
with a benign but rapidly progressive BPH may suffer
bladder-neck obstruction, followed by infection of
the ureters and kidneys, that could prove fatal within
a year or two, whereas an older man with virtually
inactive Stage A-1 cancer may go untreated but remain free of symptoms for the rest of his life.

The greatest uncertainty is in relation to Stage A,
Grade 2, and its likely progression to Stage B. For a
cancer still technically Stage A but rated Grade 2,
because it is larger and perhaps also more diffuse,
many (perhaps most) urologists will recommend a
prostatectomy. This may be a retropubic, as described in Chapter Eight, not of the most radical
type, and need not necessarily induce impotence although it will certainly make the patient infertile.
(This last effect may be academic, not only because
of the patient's advanced age, but because in virtually all prostatectomies the surgeons must perform a
simultaneous bilateral vasectomy. (This is not for

medical reasons, but because of the close physical relationship between the vas and the prostate.)

But for Stage A-2 patients and for some with later-stage disease there is now the option of radiation treatment. One of the earliest practitioners of this method, if not its originator, was Dr. Rubin H. Flocks of the University of Iowa, who reported in 1964 on his results in treating Stage C adenocarcinoma by injecting a solution containing radioactive gold (Au-198). The use of radioisotopes in the treatment of various solid tumors is, of course, much older. Gold pellets containing "radium" (actually its gaseous daughter, radon) were in wide use shortly after World War II. One of the questions to be resolved in deciding upon a radioisotope suitable for implantation is the "hardness" or "softness" of the rays emitted by the element, as this largely determines how far they will travel. If their range extends too far, they will damage healthy tissues. Another factor in the choice of an isotope is how long the radioactivity will persist.

At Memorial, Dr. Whitmore decided that for relatively early prostatic cancer the most suitable radiation source is one of the several isotopes of iodine, specifically I-125. This is a soft gamma emitter, so the rays (more precisely, subatomic particles) do not travel too far, and it loses half its strength every sixty days. With the patient anesthetized, a physician inserts thin metal tubes through the pubic region into the prostate. Then, through these tubes, he propels tiny pellets of titanium covered with gold and containing Iodine-125. The pellets are only 4.75 mm. (less than 1/5 in.) long and .75 mm. (about 1/32 in.) in diameter. At the end of two months the patient's prostate has received 8,000 rads, which would be a heavy dose if it were not so carefully localized. At the end of a year the prostate has received a cumulative total of about 16,000 rads, but the radioactivity has reached a level so low as to be negligible. The pellets, too small to cause any discomfort and now essentially inert, can safely remain in the patient's prostate for the rest of his life. The implants have no effect on a man's sexual potency, and patients needing this type of treatment are almost always of an age at which they should no longer be worried about fertility.

An alternative to internal irradiation from implanted sources is external radiation. This is appropriate for patients whose disease is still in Stage A but rated Grade 2 and unlikely to be cured by a TUR because the cancer either has formed at several points or is diffuse in nature. External radiation may also be chosen as the primary treatment for many cases of Stage B and as additional therapy for some patients with later-stage disease.

The external radiation technique has been developed principally by Dr. Malcolm A. Bagshaw, of Stanford University, who is its most vocal advocate and has treated Rogers C. B. Morton, the first prominent personality to acknowledge his prostatic disease publicly. In the selection of a patient for external radiation treatment there are two basic considerations, one positive, one negative: 1) he must be in good enough general physical condition to tolerate heavy doses of high-energy radiation delivered during a short time but repeated four or five days a week for several (usually seven) weeks, and 2) he must not have Stage D cancer that has metastatized to parts of the body remote from the prostate. To produce the type of radiation required, extremely high voltages delivering high-energy particles are necessary. Several devices are capable of doing this, but the two most commonly used are a cobalt-60 source and the linear accelerator.

Dr. Bagshaw was the first physician to put the linear accelerator to medical use in the United States, employing Stanford's machine for this purpose in 1956. He still prefers it to any other, on the ground that its high-energy beam can be focused more sharply than those from other sources, meaning that it does less damage to surrounding tissues, and that the rays can be made to stop more precisely at the desired depth. However, at a satellite clinic operated by Stanford, where a linear accelerator is not available, he is satisfied to use a cobalt-60 source.

In 1974 the wives of both President Gerald Ford and Vice President Nelson Rockefeller had radical mastectomies for breast cancer. They were by far the most prominent patients to allow widespread and detailed publicity about their condition and resulting operations. But a year earlier a public figure in his own right had let it be known that he had been diagnosed as having cancer of the prostate and had undergone treatment for it. It is symptomatic of the difference in public attitudes toward female breast disease and male prostate disease that the man's case attracted minimal attention.

Rogers Morton was fifty-eight years old and Secretary of the Interior in February 1973, when probable cancer of the prostate was detected during a routine physical examination. (Morton had not been aware of any symptoms.) Further tests confirmed the diagnosis of what Morton's press secretary called an "early-stage malignancy." The exact stage was not disclosed, but the treatment indicates that Morton's cannot have been an earliest, Stage A-1 case.

Morton was offered the choice between a prostatectomy, with no guarantee that a slight spread of the malignancy beyond the prostate capsule would be entirely removed, or the radiation treatment developed by Dr. Bagshaw. Morton decided on the latter and spent seven weeks in and near Stanford, visiting the hospital five days a week except for alternate Wednesdays off. Morton's body was aligned under Stanford's 4.8 million volt linear accelerator and its beam was focused first on his prostate. On each day of treatment he received a radiation dose of 220 rads, most of it directed to the prostate—but not all.

Despite some continuing controversy as to whether the prostate is endowed with ducts for the circulation of lymphatic fluid (in addition to its self-evident blood supply), Dr. Bagshaw believes that one way for a cancer originating in the prostate to spread and colonize other parts of the body is through the lymph nodes in the pelvis. (The pelvis is that part of the trunk below the abdomen; it can usually be considered as beginning a couple of inches below the navel.) So some of those 220 rads are directed higher, focused on the pelvic nodes, in the hope of protecting them against any wandering cancerous cells. The method is called "extended-field therapy."

At the end of the Secretary's seven-week stint, Dr. Bagshaw noted that he had responded well to the treatment, and added, "There is every reason to be optimistic about his condition." More than three years later that optimism appeared thoroughly justified. While Morton remained as Secretary of the Interior, members of his staff said that he continued to "run the feet off" subordinates half his age; thrice weekly he went to Interior's gym for an hour and a half of hard-played handball.

Morton later changed jobs, but not to accept a lighter one. Instead, he assumed what were probably more demanding duties for President Ford. The case history of Rogers Morton clearly shows that prostatic cancer, detected relatively early and treated expertly, is far from being a sentence of imminent disablement or death.

Morton's case is notable because he is a public figure, but it is typical of hundreds that Dr. Bagshaw and his associates have treated since 1956. No fewer than 72 percent of patients with disease limited to the prostate have survived five years (66 percent with no recurrence of disease and no need for additional treatment such as the administration of hormones), and 44 percent have survived ten years. For patients whose disease extended beyond the prostatic capsule at the time of diagnosis and treatment, the survival rate was 51 percent after five years and 38 percent after ten years. The Stanford results are beyond question extraordinarily good. Whether they are superior to those at other centers with equally expert physicians may not be proved until prostate cancer detection and treatment are better standardized.

For Stage B and the more advanced stages, Dr. Gerald P. Murphy, Director of the Roswell Park Memorial Institute and also of the National Prostatic Cancer Project, has devised a sophisticated system of grading cancers by the tissues and cells that are successively involved. The details are extremely technical,* but the grade of the primary tumor at its original site appears to be well correlated with at least two important biochemical variables and with patients' responses to selected treatments. Extended from the research-testing stage to the treatment of patients, this information should, in the near future, enable doctors to select treatment methods and medications on a far more certain basis than at present.

Once a patient has Stage B cancer, some type of prostatectomy is almost although no longer absolutely mandatory. In the more severe cases (which may be a majority today, because of delays in detection), it will be a radical, retropubic or perineal op-

---

* The commonly held concept of cancer as a disease caused by cells multiplying too rapidly is an oversimplification. It is true that they may multiply rapidly, but the most important aspect of their behavior is that they do not mature (technically, "differentiate") so as to function like normal, fully developed cells. They continue to multiply needlessly, crowding out the remaining normal cells and eventually entire organ masses.

eration, if not a total. For Stage C it will be a truly total operation. The distinction between the different forms of "radical" prostatectomy and the "total" is that in the former the capsule of the gland is not removed, although its contents are emptied to varying degrees, whereas in the latter the entire capsule is cut out. This necessarily means sacrificing many of the nerves and muscle connections between the gland, the bladder neck, and the urethra. In consequence, the patient will be impotent, with no possibility of attaining an erection. He may also suffer incontinence after his recovery from the surgery.

Cancer specialists still have in reserve several more drastic measures designed primarily to prolong the life of the patient. Only in a minority of cases do these advanced treatments restore the patients to full comfort, but the majority are grateful for the prolongation of life with some relief of symptoms.

If we date radical prostatectomies from about 1890, then fifty years passed before the next major advance. This, ironically, was a revival of the ancient practice of subtotal castration. The procedure does not involve any operation on the penis, a fact that needs to be emphasized because suprisingly many men are confused and therefore unduly fearful when this surgery is suggested to them. Because it involves removal of the testicles, surgeons prefer to call the procedure "bilateral orchiectomy" or "orchidectomy." (*Orchis* is the Greek word both for the testicle and for a ground orchid with a tuberous root of the same shape.)

Dr. Charles B. Huggins of the University of Chicago, with the essential help of a third-year medical student, Clarence V. Hodges, discovered in 1940 that prostate cancer was largely under the control of the sex hormones: androgens (male hormones, mainly testosterone) promoted its growth, while estrogens (female hormones) retarded it.

To leave the prostate a sharply reduced supply of testosterone, which is secreted mainly in the testicles, Dr. Huggins proposed to castrate the patients. Some, despite their advanced years, refused the surgery, rating the treatment worse than their disease. Such refusals were based largely on the mistaken belief that castration would leave them with feminine voices and conspicuous breasts. (The fact is that these effects of castration do not occur in men beyond middle age, although the breasts of some older men become enlarged naturally—the condition called gynecomastia. These changes occur without any surgical or medical intervention.) Some of the patients in their sixties and seventies refused the operation because it would make them sterile, although they could offer no valid reason for desiring continued fertility.

With so few takers for his surgical procedure, Dr. Huggins turned to a medicinal alternative: administration of the female hormone, diethylstilbestrol (DES). Taking a white pill was naturally far more acceptable to greater numbers of patients. There is no proof that either orchiectomy or hormone treatment has ever cured a case of Stage C or D cancer, but both procedures have prolonged lives and made these lives more comfortable. In 1966, Dr. Huggins belatedly received a Nobel Prize for his accomplishment; unaccountably, Dr. Hodges did not share in the award.

One peculiarity of hormonal treatment for prostate cancer is that if the disease is well controlled for a while by the administration of oral DES, and this treatment later loses its effectiveness, a substantial number of patients can then gain a new lease on life from castration. For reasons not yet known, the converse is not true.

Encouraged by the success of the Huggins procedures, other investigators began to study the possibility of still more hormonal intervention. The first, and perhaps the most obvious, was to remove the adrenal glands, because these secrete a modest amount of testosterone. The relative lack of success of this procedure results from the fact that the adrenals do not secrete sufficient testosterone for their removal to make a significant difference in the life prospects of any considerable number of patients.

Since the adrenals, like the testicles, are under the control of master hormones produced in the pituitary gland, or "hypophysis," the next and more radical hormonal intervention consisted of the removal of this gland. This is surgically a most difficult procedure, since the pituitary is concealed in the middle of the skull, inside a bony structure which serves it as a bomb shelter. At least three different approaches to the pituitary to permit its removal have been devised. But the risks of this surgery, and possible side effects because other hormonal mechanisms are interfered with, suggest that hypophysectomy is unlikely to be accepted as a common procedure.

In the search for methods of checking the stimulating effect of testosterone on the prostate, various hormone-blocking agents have been tested. One of the first was cyproterone acetate, which can be taken conveniently by mouth. Unfortunately, it was found that cyproterone acetate not only blocks testosterone metabolism but overreaches its desired effects and interferes with many other of the body's metabolic processes, including those involving cholesterol. It has now been dropped as a treatment for prostatic cancer, but other metabolic blockers are being investigated. The most promising at this writing is Flutamide (also known by its manufacturer's designation, SCH. 13521). This appears to be at least as effective for most patients as the female hormone DES, and to have the advantage of sparing younger patients the feminizing side effects of DES. About 25 percent of patients who failed, initially or later, to respond to DES have been reported to respond favorably to Flutamide, and it is reasonable to expect that more potent hormone-modifying medications will be developed in the near future.

With the addition of chemotherapy—the use of synthetic medications not related to the body's natural hormones—there are now at least five different kinds of treatment for prostatic cancer: 1) a TUR for an evidently small and localized lesion in its earliest stages; 2) prostatectomies of varying degrees, up to the total removal of the gland and adjacent structures; 3) radiation, both internal and external; 4) hormonal manipulation by surgery (orchiectomy, adrenalectomy, hypophysectomy) or administration of female hormones or "antiandrogens," and 5) chemotherapy.

During this century investigative emphasis has changed from the various forms of prostatectomy to almost as many forms of hormonal manipulation, to radiation (still largely neglected in many medical centers), to chemotherapy. At present, concentration on the hormonal approach has given way to intensified efforts to find the most effective biochemical treatments with the fewest and least distressing side effects.

To be effective against cancer cells, a medicinal chemical or "chemotherapeutic agent" must interfere with the metabolism of the cells. The most sensitive point in the chain at which metabolism and therefore growth and multiplication can be interrupted involves the stage at which folic acid is taken up. This has already been discussed in connection with the uptake and use of folic acid by bacteria, which can be inhibited by trimethoprim (see Chapter Six). But trimethoprim has no effect on the metabolism of human cells. In the treatment of cancers, the chemotherapeutist is confronted with a dilemma: he wishes to block the metabolism of the abnormal, cancerous cells, while sparing the normal cells. But there is a very fine line between the metabolic processes of the normal and the cancerous cells, so that any medication that blocks the metabolism and therefore the multiplication of cancerous cells is likely to have some of the same effect, although, it is hoped, to a less degree, upon normal cells.

In 1957 two potent antifolic medications were developed: cyclophosphamide, perhaps better known by its trade name of Cytoxan, and 5-fluorouracil, usually abbreviated to 5-FU. These soon proved their effectiveness against several forms of cancer, but either were not tried, or were not used in the most appropriate manner, against cancer of the prostate until recently. Cytoxan has proved most effective against malignant diseases of the lymphatic system and some forms of leukemia; it has been found less effective against solid tumors—including, somewhat surprisingly, carcinoma of the breast, whose tissues are similar in many respects to those of the prostate. Its manufacturers recommend that it be employed against prostatic cancer only by physicians who are especially well versed in dealing with its possible and indeed, probable unfavorable side effects. Roche Laboratories, the manufacturers of 5-FU, go even farther: they recommend that it be given only under the supervision of a highly qualified physician, and further, that all patients receiving it be hospitalized at least during the early stages of treatment.

Despite these major disadvantages, Cytoxan and 5-FU have now been shown, if not to retard the advance of metastatic cancer originating in the prostate, at least to mitigate many of its symptoms.

More recently still, a noxious agent has been found, in a new combination, to have similar palliative although not curative effects in advanced prostate cancer. This is one of the nitrogen mustards, a derivative of the mustard gas that was developed during World War I. Laboratory refinements produced still more potent forms of the basic substance during World War II, but these, mercifully, were not used in warfare as far as is known. Now one of the nitrogen mustards has been combined with an estrogen in a formulation called Estracyt, which seems to have inhibitory effects upon the spread of metastasizing prostatic cancer, or at least to reduce patient discomfort.

Combinations of all these medications are being used with increasing optimism in the treatment of advanced prostatic cancer, and in addition Dr. Murphy reports that under the auspices of the National Prostatic Cancer Project at least six other agents of possible value are being tested in a number of cancer centers.

The current emphasis on chemotherapy may prove to be excessive in itself, as well as the subject of excessive optimism by its advocates. The one thing on which every specialist in the field agrees—with the possible exception of a few who may have a vested interest in one particular form of treatment—is that far too little is yet known about the origins of benign prostatic overgrowth, let alone about the initiation of cancer and its progression from the prostate to adjacent and eventually to remote organs. To achieve the necessary greater understanding of these fundamental processes, urologists and cancer specialists must go back to the geneticists and immunologists for investigations that will probe the observed phenomena at a far deeper level than has yet been reached.

At present the emphasis is largely upon the treatment of advanced disease. As Dr. Whitmore says, "The therapy of prostatic cancer is extremely controversial, and legitimately so. We would all like to have much more information on the basis of which we could resolve these controversies. We know that because cancer of the prostate is a disease principally of older men, there is a substantial mortality from other causes—in fact this may reach 85 to 90 percent. The mortality from cancer, in patients with locally extensive but not metastatic disease, is only about 25 percent at most. With metastases, the mortality from cancer increases to about 50 percent, but that is not until you are dealing with Stage D cancer.

"But there are exceptions—you can't generalize—because the natural course of the disease is totally unpredictable and extremely variable in both its patterns and its rates of progression. The younger the patient is, the worse the prognosis. Yet a man at the age of sixty with Stage B prostatic cancer may refuse surgery and still live to a ripe old age. It is impossible to assemble valid comparative data for patients treated at different centers, because the selection of those who will receive treatment by different methods varies so widely. We cannot compare patients treated by radical prostatectomy with those treated by our radioactive implants because the criteria for selection are so different. You cannot even compare our implant patients with those treated by external radiation.

"In sum, the impact of any treatment is uncertain. In any large number of patients you do not know what percentage will respond well and have long survivals and what percentage will not—and even if you knew that you could still not predict the category into which any particular patient would fall. We believe that our patients with the radiation implants have as much benefit from this procedure as those treated in other ways and that they suffer fewer adverse effects on urination, and on bowel and sexual function. You might say that we think they are getting as good a product at a lower physiological price. But so much remains to be learned that we simply remain humble in the face of the unknown."

Dr. Murphy, of the National Prostatic Cancer Project, complains that many urologists and urologic surgeons, adherents of different schools, may talk to each other but either do not listen or are not receptive. A further difficulty of this type is that urologists and radiologists, in Dr. Murphy's words, "tend not to speak each other's language." One of his major concerns is to improve communication between specialists and subspecialists in all fields related to prostate cancer. From this, he believes, must come greater cooperation and a sharing of research knowledge and therapeutic experience—all to be applied for the benefit of the patient.

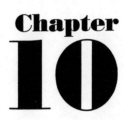

Chapter 10

Psyche and Eros

One of the most unfortunate aspects of prostatic disorder, however mild it may be, is that in the vast majority of cases it attacks men at a time of life when they are least equipped either physically or psychologically to cope with the problem. The slightest disturbance of urinary function raises questions that the average layman is totally unable to answer. He wonders whether he is beginning to undergo what has been overpublicized as the male climacteric. If there really is such a thing as a male climacteric, it has yet to be precisely defined, and the one thing certain about it is that it bears little or no resemblance to the female climacteric or menopause.

At some time in her life, commonly in the years just before or about the age of fifty, a woman undergoes a fairly precise and certainly definable physiological and biochemical change. She ceases to secrete as much estrogen as before. Over a period that may extend from three months to three or four years, the processes of both ovulation and menstruation come to an end. This has been recognized for thousands of years, even though precise biochemical measurements of the hormonal changes have been possible only in recent decades. Accompanying these changes there is sometimes a marked temperamental crisis, in which a woman becomes irritable, edgy, and intolerant of petty details that she would formerly have ignored. This phenomenon, both during the menopause and in the years following it, is so pronounced that some pharmaceutical manufacturers market tranquilizers solely on the basis of experience with their use by postmenopausal women.

At about the same age men may become equally irritable, edgy, and intolerant of petty details, but in their case there is no comparable biochemical explanation. There is no male climacteric in which the production of an important sexual hormone declines abruptly, and there are no changes in the male comparable with the cessation of ovulation and menstruation in the female. The only change in the male that is even roughly comparable is some decrease in the activity of testosterone. This is not explainable on the basis of a simple decline in the amount of testosterone secreted by the testicles and the adrenal glands. There is commonly some such decrease, but it is not consistent, and whatever changes in the male's sexual interests and activities are associated with it seem more likely to derive from alterations in the metabolism of testosterone. These alterations are currently the subject of research by a number of urologists and sexologists, but as yet there is no consensus as to how extensive they are, or just what their nature and effects may be.

But men are faced with changes of many kinds,

usually beginning in the late forties but often not noticeable until the mid-fifties. These changes result from several factors that may simply happen to coincide in time. Most men of fifty have reached the apex of their careers. A few, especially in the upper echelons of big business and certain professions, may go on to greater achievements that carry with them enormous satisfactions, but these are a minority. Some men accept the idea of having reached a plateau in their careers, take it with good grace, and remain calm and well balanced. A substantial number, however, feel that they face a barrier that they cannot surmount, and are rebellious and depressed. So we observe simultaneously a gradual natural decline in physical energy and, perhaps, a more abrupt decline in ambition or of confidence in accomplishment. When this happens to a man in his fifties it is glibly said that he is undergoing the male climacteric. By the time he is seventy, if the same changes are still more evident, everybody says, "Oh, it's old age that's getting him down." For twenty years Dr. Harold A. Lear practiced urology in Connecticut; then he took specialized psychiatric training and developed the Human Sexuality Program at the Mount Sinai Medical Center in New York. He says that in some ways the use of the term "male climacteric" is nothing more or less than putting a dramatic label on a natural phase of life.

Dr. Lear points out that the often reported, and perhaps overemphasized, changes in testosterone secretion that accompany the aging process are much less pronounced than those that occur in a normal younger man's life within any twenty-four-hour period. For example, there are great variations in testosterone secretion from well below normal to tremendous highs that occur within a minute or two during sleep. These changes have not been correlated with the depth-of-sleep cycle or with dreaming. There is also a cycle during the day's working hours, with testosterone levels highest in the morning. These normal ups and downs around the clock involve blood-stream concentrations of testosterone varying by a factor of ten or twenty or even more—far greater than the diminishing factor attributed to aging.

Although the roller-coaster levels of testosterone are not fully understood, they are known to be related to both libido and sexual ability. But they cannot be directly related to sexual stimulation or charged with total responsibility for whatever differences a man is aware of in these aspects of his life pattern, because there are so many other factors that must be considered. One of the most important, to which little formal attention has been paid, is the feedback effect upon a man of the changes in women's reactions to him, especially the reactions of women younger than himself.

Just when he is beset by the elements in his social and working life that cause self-doubt, a man is most likely to become aware of symptoms of prostate disorder. Almost invariably the first symptom is having to get up in the middle of the night to urinate. This nocturia is simply a sign of a mild and gradual benign prostatic hypertrophy, in which the lateral and anterior lobes of the prostate are the ones most likely to enlarge. They are also the ones that encroach upon the urethra. Nocturia is not necessarily related to the *extent* of BPH; it depends largely on the *degree* of constriction that the enlargement imposes upon the urethra. Since this type of benign enlargement rarely involves the posterior lobe, the prostate may feel completely normal to the physician performing the rectal examination, while it nevertheless causes considerable squeezing of the urinary passage. The narrowing of the urethra may lead to frequency and urgency of nocturnal voiding because of either incomplete emptying of the bladder or an irritative reaction in the part of the urethra immediately below the bladder.

A man entering his fifties is likely to exacerbate this problem by consuming more alcoholic drinks and coffee, both of which act as diuretics. His intake of these beverages is related both to his gradual change in life style and to an increasingly pronounced reaction to stress. Although there are scores of highly technical medical works on the subject of stress, no one yet has been able to offer a satisfactory definition of it in lay terms. For our purposes, the best definition may be utterly unscientific but intensely practical: a man is suffering from stress when he gets the feeling that "Everything is too much for me." He may have financial difficulties, aggravated by a career impasse. He may have teenage or young adult offspring who are creating problems. And at this time in a man's life he is likely to have a menopausal wife with her own worries and difficulties.

When he goes to sleep (with or without the help of a pill) he is far from relaxed. His emotional tension alone may be enough to wake him after four or five hours, so that he then needs to get up and urinate. If he were truly relaxed, he might sleep seven or eight hours without this need. But in all likelihood he will not relate his nocturia to his emotional stress. It is easier and less disturbing to blame physical rather than psychological factors.

Urinary urgency and frequency may result as much or more from stress as from physiological changes. No sharp line can be drawn between the two contributing factors.

At the very time of life when it is least desirable, medically speaking, for a man to do so, he is likely to develop a preference for highly spiced foods. This is because he is losing some of his taste buds. Hot peppers and curry, no matter how well they stimulate a jaded appetite, have diuretic and often irritative effects upon the urinary tract. Another common cause of nocturia or of urgency and frequency is cystitis, a mild infection of the bladder. When this is diagnosed it can be treated simply and effectively with a ten-day course of one of the familiar sulfas.

The layman cannot diagnose his own urinary disorders or determine whether they are related to the prostate. The clear warning signals that should send any sensible man to a doctor include: a need to urinate that reaches a frequency such as four times a night; difficulty in either starting to urinate or maintaining a strong and steady stream; a burning sensation after urination or a dribbling after it appears to have been completed. Of course any sign of blood in the urine, or any other notable discoloration, should similarly propel him toward his family doctor or a urologist. After listening to a recital of the standard symptoms, the urologist will run laboratory tests and X rays, and may recommend medication, or surgery such as a TUR for BPH.

It is often assumed that if a man undergoes even this relatively untraumatic procedure for prostatic disorder he is likely to have resulting problems in his sexual life. Dr. Lear says this is not necessarily true. There is, he maintains, no simple one-to-one correlation between the surgical procedure and sexual performance or ability. There are too many variables. Many men function normally and with no complaints in their sex life after a TUR or other prostatic surgery. Whether the operation consists of a suprapubic or retropubic prostatectomy makes no difference to the man's ability to have sexual relations. The one procedure that almost invariably produces impotence is the total (usually perineal) prostatectomy, because in this the nerve and muscle connections to the urethra, which control the erectile process, are surgically severed.

Otherwise, the number of prostate operations that result in impotence is remarkably small. After a TUR, only fourteen out of a hundred men who were formerly sexually potent complain of impotence, says Dr. Lear. And it is uncertain how many of the few who become impotent do so because of a physiological change resulting from the surgery. Present-day research indicates that the cause is more likely to be psychological, the result of poor counseling and insufficient understanding of the operation. For men who have suprapubic or retropubic prostatectomies, the incidence of impotence following surgery runs as high as 20 to 25 percent, but no higher. In such cases it is possible that some of the nerve and muscle connections needed for penile erection have been damaged in surgery, but again, psychological factors probably play a role in many instances.

A key factor in answering the question whether prostate surgery impairs a man's sexual function is to be found in comparing his description of his pattern of sexual behavior, which should be conscientiously recorded by the doctor before surgery, with his complaint of impotence after the operation. In a surprising number of cases the man who asserts that his private life has been ruined by his operation will be found, when the record is checked, to have stated well before the operation that he was already impotent.

If there is any impairment of sexual function following the more common forms of prostatic surgery, it may well result from something as simple as a man's ignorance of the significance of the procedure. An astonishing number of intelligent adult males simply do not know the difference between potency and fertility. As a result, they tend—perhaps unconsciously—to equate any form of prostatic surgery with castration or at least with demasculination. Unless they are adequately counseled in advance of surgery, which unfortunately is an uncommon part of the urologist's performance, these men are likely to have self-fulfilling prophetic ideas about the effects their operations will have. If the urologist has neither the time nor the training to counsel his patients adequately, he should refer them to a specialist in this type of practice.

There is a reverse side to this coin: other men, but perhaps a minority, become determined to prove after surgery that they are still sexually competent, and they may achieve greater activity.

The one indisputable physiological effect of any prostatic surgery other than a TUR is that, as mentioned earlier, after the operation a man will have no discernible ejaculation at orgasm. This results from the fact that of the two sphincters controlling the urethra to prevent urination during sexual excitation and to permit erection, the lower sphincter remains closed, so that erection is still possible. But the upper sphincter leading from the bladder to the urethra is open because its nerve-muscle connections have been cut. The result is that the output of the ejaculatory ducts in the prostate is discharged into the upper urethra by what is called retrograde ejaculation. The material enters the bladder, from which it is expelled at the next urination, mixed with urine and unnoticed.

The physical effects of prostatic surgery must be carefully considered, but their importance tends to be overemphasized. The comparable effects of the psyche upon Eros may be still greater, but are too often underrated. If a man goes into the operating room well informed and adequately counseled, he is likely soon to be as sexually proficient as he was before the operation—and thanks to the relief of painful symptoms, the experience may be considerably more satisfying to both partners.

Chapter

Looking Ahead

Advances beyond those already achieved in the control and cure of disorders of the prostate, ranging from the mildest urinary disturbance to cancer, must be based upon continuing and intensified medical research along two principal pathways. The one that has attracted the greater amount of attention from investigators, because it involves so many men with crippling and painful disease, concerns measures against cancer. This, necessarily, is applied medical science, and it is understandable that it must be the course of primary effort at this time.

However, truly basic research into the nature of the changes that occur in the prostate is essential to a better understanding of the gland's numerous functions, and without such understanding there can be little hope of prevention of any of the disorders. In effect, research effort has been directed backward from the case of the patient with Stage D cancer that has already spread to other organs and is essentially incurable, to the earliest stages of the same disease. Dr. Murphy, director of the National Prostatic Cancer Project, is extremely enthusiastic about the recent developments in chemotherapy, some of which have been discussed in a previous chapter. He notes that the plight of the late-stage victim of prostatic cancer can be markedly eased with the administration of Cytoxan and 5-FU. "The important thing," Dr. Murphy says, "is that we have just shown that these agents will still work for many patients who have already had everything else—castration, hormone therapy, radiation—the works. They are best of all for relieving pain."

The investigation of chemical agents or synthetic medications for relief of the distressing symptoms of prostatic cancer has been extraordinarily slow in development. Dr. Joseph B. Schmidt, of the University of Iowa group of urologic specialists, uses the expression "woefully neglected." As recently as the end of 1974, he reports, only about 10 percent of the available anticancer drugs had been tested against prostatic adenocarcinoma, whereas some 90 percent had been tested against the two other most frequent solid tumors afflicting men, colon and lung cancer. Dr. Schmidt understands that it is natural to use these potent chemicals in the hope of relieving the distress of patients in late stages of the disease, but he contends that it would be more rational in terms of the greatest good for the greatest number to try using these drugs along with surgery or radiation at earlier stages of the disease, to see whether they will retard the growth of a tumor.

Some anticancer medications work best when the cells are dividing and going through the process of

DNA synthesis. One such is 5-FU. Other agents are effective regardless of the stage in the cells' reproductive cycle at which they are administered. So it is logical, says Dr. Schmidt, to combine treatment with one of each type. This, he believes, may even reduce the "tumor burden" on the patient to the extent that his own immune mechanisms will have sufficient strength to kill the remainder of the malignant cells.

Of the newer anticancer medications now being extensively tested, the most promising appear to be Estracyt—the combination of a nitrogen mustard derivative with an estrogen—and streptozotocin. The former has the advantage of being administered orally; the latter is injected intravenously. Streptozotocin is a modified antibiotic; the only other antibiotic of any significant value against prostatic cancer is adriamycin. At least half a dozen other medications, some entirely synthetic and others semisynthetic, are being tested against prostate cancer. Some of them are already being used in the treatment of human patients; others are still in the animal experiment stage.

Dr. Murphy says: "We still have no cure for the disease, except in cases that are detected very early, and these are distressingly few. Just as in the case of breast cancer, prostate specialists argue vehemently about every aspect of treatment for the disease, whether surgical or other. However, I feel that having disagreement over several available treatments is far better than having no treatment, which was the case within the lifetime of virtually every investigator now working on the disease. Not only are we getting new drugs of different types, but we are doing comparative studies on their effects."

Dr. Murphy properly and understandably insists that the prospects for effective treatment will be enormously improved if men will take the simple, self-protective step of submitting themselves for physical, including rectal, examinations beginning in earlier decades of their life, and have the examinations repeated more frequently as they get older. The fact that fewer than 5 percent of the 250,000 prostatectomies performed annually in the United States are for cancer appears at first glance to be encouraging. But this is deceptive: if a greater proportion of the operations were for cancer, it would mean that more men were having the disease diagnosed at an early and curable stage.

Some investigators, emphasizing the need for prevention of prostatic cancer, have reported an increased incidence of cervical and uterine cancer in their patients' wives. This is a preliminary finding and has yet to be confirmed. There is, on the other hand, the possibility of a beneficial male-female crossover in relation to prostatitis: both gynecologists and urologists are being urged to pay more attention to women's vestigial prostatic tissue, hitherto neglected, as a source of urinary difficulties.

Basic research into the nature of prostatic disorders is hampered by the fact that, with the possible exception of the baboon, there is no animal in which a disease comparable with the human form can be studied. It is further hampered by the fact that prostate cells cannot yet be grown in laboratory glassware for more than one generation. This is in sharp contrast with certain other types of human cells which have been kept reproducing under artificial conditions outside the body for at least one human generation and for hundreds of cell generations.

Dr. Aaron Bendich, of the Sloan-Kettering Institute for Cancer Research, is especially concerned about this difficulty, because he has been studying the effects of spermatozoa upon normal prostatic cells. He points out that the anatomy of the prostate was not adequately worked out and described until the early 1970s, and that the old textbooks' treatment of the subject is at best uninformative and at worst misleading. Dr. Bendich puts considerable emphasis on the extreme activity of several internal structures during sexual intercourse which climaxes, of course, at orgasm. At this time, he believes, fluid is forced back up through the urethra in the region of the verumontanum and therefore can enter the prostatic ducts. Sometimes spermatozoa may be forced back into the ducts in this way. Because many of the changes that are produced in normal cells by cancer-causing chemicals are also produced by spermatozoa, the suspicion arises that the backward-flowing sperm may be involved in the initiation of prostatic cancer. So far, however, it has not been possible to culture prostatic cells well enough to prove that this phenomenon occurs in the human male. Dr. Bendich is one of those who believe that benign prostatic hypertrophy may be a natural process in the mature man. But then, for cancer to develop, there must be a promoter of abnormal cellular growth, and up to now no such promoter has been identified.

Another approach to prostatic cancer has been initiated by Dr. George C. Cotzias, also of Sloan-Kettering. Dr. Cotzias is the physician who developed the first effective treatment for Parkinsonism, through the administration of what were at first considered massive doses of L-Dopa, a metabolic precursor that the brain uses as raw material from which to manufacture dopamine. Its benefit in Parkinson's disease results from the fact that it enables the brain to correct a dopamine deficiency. The connection between this and prostatic cancer may seem remote, but Dr. Cotzias' interest was aroused by another investigator's report that L-Dopa appeared to have pain-killing effects in some forms of cancer. Again it was found that heavier dosages than would normally be considered advisable had to be used. Dr. Cotzias was further intrigued by the fact that a pain-killing effect was observed in patients suffering from breast cancer, but not in those having cancer of the colon.

Dr. Cotzias' own investigations showed him that in every case in which he treated an animal with an anticancer medication there was some effect on the dopamine content of the brain. But the effect was not the same with different types of medications: those of natural biological origin improved the communication between brain cells, whereas the synthetic chemical agents inhibited it. Pursuing this clue, Dr. Cotzias and his colleagues found that one strain of laboratory mice in which the females have an extraordinarily strong tendency to develop spontaneous breast cancer had the lowest concentration of dopamine in their brains. On the other hand, females of a strain with a negligible tendency to develop breast cancer had the highest concentration. It therefore appears that something in the brains of these animals, something genetically determined, correlates with the tendency to develop breast cancer. Since the equivalent of female breast tissue is that of the prostate in the male, Dr. Cotzias' group is now testing biological materials in the treatment of patients with advanced disease.

Another major line of attack against the development and progression of cancer is through the human system's natural defense mechanisms. These consist primarily of immune reactions, and some investigators hope and believe that these reactions can be stimulated to perform more effectively if the patients are treated with BCG, the antituberculosis vaccine. It is known also that there is a bactericidal (bacteria-killing) substance in the prostate. Just what it is no one yet knows, and it is obvious that whatever it is, it is often of low potency. Conceivably a way to reinforce this substance can be found.

The result of these various research efforts should be not only palliation or even cure of life-threatening prostatic disease, but eventually the prevention of benign hypertrophy.

The prostate, whose very existence went unrecognized for so long, will remain forever hidden in the pelvic cavity. But although the gland remains physically hidden, it has at last emerged into public as well as medical awareness as an organ that can be openly discussed. This had to happen before it could become the subject of extensive, planned medical research. The prostate is important in procreation, sexual fulfillment, and marital happiness. Its vital role in the health of millions of men entitles it to the recognition and research attention that it is now at last receiving, and which should be increased.

Index